CURING CHRONIC ILLNESS
(Mental or Physical)
The Diet Solution

Alan Hunter Ph.D (A.M.)
Award-winning author of
Curing Food Allergies

Bright Pen

A Bright Pen Book

British Library Cataloguing Publication Data.
A catalogue record for this book is available from the British Library

ISBN 978-0-7552-0740-4

Authors OnLine Ltd
19 The Cinques
Gamlingay, Sandy
Bedfordshire SG19 3NU
England

This book is also available in e-book format, details of which are available at
www.authorsonline.co.uk

DISCLAIMER

While the author of this book has made every effort to ensure that the information contained in this book is as accurate and up-to-date as possible at the time of publication, medical and pharmaceutical knowledge is constantly changing and the application of it to particular circumstances depends on many factors. This book should not be used as an alternative to specialised medical advice and it is recommended that readers always consult a qualified health professional for individual advice before following any new diet or health programme. The author and publishers cannot be held responsible for any errors and omissions that may be found in the text, or any actions that may be taken by a reader, as a result of any reliance on the information contained in the text, which are taken entirely at the reader's own risk. The contents are not intended to treat, diagnose or prevent any disease.

ACKNOWLEDGEMENTS

I wish to thank the following, either for their direct or indirect contributions to this book or for their influence their work has had on my views on the causes of illness:

Charlotte Gerson, of the world-famous Gerson Institute in California, for allowing me access to many case histories of recovered patients; Dr. Herbert Shelton and Dr. George Clements, for their wonderful books on Natural Hygiene and Orthopathy; Arnold de Vries, for his works on primitive diets, and Dr. Christine Nolfi and Dr. Wong Hon Sun, for their reports on their own successful battles with cancer. The hugely important works of Dr. Francis Pottenger, Sir Robert McCarrison, and Weston A. Price must also be acknowledged. Thanks also to Cary Mosier of Cafe Gratitude in Los Angeles.

IMPORTANT

The information in this book is intended primarily for those sufferers of illness who have been diagnosed by their doctor, but, despite medications, are still troubled by their illness. In other words, the main, presenting symptom has not been completely *cured*. If you are taking medication and the symptoms return when you cease taking them, then clearly no actual *cure* has been found for your condition. This book is based on research by the author and is not intended as a substitute for consulting with your doctor. Any attempt to diagnose or treat an illness should be done under the guidance of a healthcare professional. You must *not* cease taking any medication prescribed by your doctor, unless it is under his guidance.

USEFUL CONTACTS

1. The Gerson Institute, PO Box 161358, San Diego, CA 92176, U.S.A. Tel: (619) 685-5353   Website: www.gerson.org

2. Dr Mercola's newsletter for excellent information on health issues. Website: www.mercola.com

3. GM Watch; their email newsletters are packed with up-to-date information on the dangers of GM foods (GMOs in U.S.A.) around the world. Highly recommended for anyone concerned with their health. Contact them at editor@gmwatch.eu.   Website: www.gmwatch.eu

4. What Doctors Don't Tell You (WDDTY). Website: www.wddty.com

5. Natural News.   Website: www.naturalnews.com

6. Natural Solutions Foundation. Important information on food issues. Highly recommended newsletters. Website: www.healthfreedomusa.org

7. Hippocrates Health Institute, West Palm Beach, Florida. Website: www.hippocratesinst.org

ABOUT THE AUTHOR

Alan Hunter developed an illness at the age of 21. A top sportsman, he had to give up his beloved sport due to the frustrating symptoms.

His doctor could provide no cure and Alan felt he had no option but to do his own research in the hope he could find the answer for himself.

Clearly, as mainstream medicine had no answer, he knew he would have to think "outside the box", and his constant searching and researching meant travelling to Nature Cure Clinics and meeting with doctors worldwide.

It was whilst he was studying nutritional medicine at the Plaskett College of Nutritional Medicine, that Alan had a "Eureka" moment, arriving at the astonishing realisation that diet, body temperature, and parasitic micro-organisms were behind his – and undoubtedly many other people's – condition.

It took him 30 years to make this discovery, which eventually led to many awards. The journey is spelled out in detail in his book *Curing Food Allergies*, and a reduced version of it is included within this book (chapter 36).

On his long hunt for the solution, Alan uncovered appalling suppression of natural cures and widespread vested-interests discrediting anything that goes against the mainstream medical paradigm.

Alan won Best Research award at the Complementary Medicine Expo in London in 2003, where his research was declared as "truly original". It has also been referred to as "highly original" by the publisher of his *Curing Food Allergies.* His research also resulted in a high honour from the Indian Board of Alternative Medicines in Kolkata in 2000, where he received the Seva Ratna award for research, along with a doctorate – a PhD in Alternative Medicines – a non-traditional doctorate accredited by the Government of India Act XXI of 1860, Literary and Scientific Institutions Act, 1854. He was also awarded 1st prize for his research by Action Against Allergy.

In this latest book, Alan has again come up with another original discovery – that just as every animal in the wild, every bird, every insect, and every fish, eats its food raw, so too was man intended to eat this way. Before fire was discovered, man did indeed eat raw. Could we have been eating wrongly for thousands of years? There is compelling evidence in this book to suggest we have. Our rapidly escalating health disorders can be down to our diet, and, by choosing one closer to nature, your body can respond with a return to health. Whether it is a fully raw, or part-raw diet, health disorders can be overcome.

Alan has written for the famous Townsend Letter for Doctors and Patients (U.S.A); Journal of Alternative and Complementary Medicine (UK), Healthy Living, Here's Health and Positive Health magazines.

CONTENTS

1.

Can Raw Food Cure Disease?

Absolutely. As far back as 1905, this report on a cure for consumption (TB) was printed in the *New York Post*. It will be referred to again later in this book.

"NEW YORK: All the prominent physicians of New York have received a circular from the New York Post-Graduate Hospital announcing the discovery of a new cure for consumption. The new remedy is the juice of raw vegetables (potatoes, carrots, celery, and the like), the dose being two ounces after meals. The statement is made that eleven patients with well-developed pulmonary tuberculosis have been absolutely cured. Fifty other patients are still under treatment and are progressing satisfactorily. The experiments have been made in the above-mentioned hospital under the direction of Dr John F. Russell, who for several years has been the principal advocate of nutrition – as opposed to medication – for the treatment of tuberculosis of the pulmonary type. It is announced that the remedy will doubtless be shortly obtainable from all chemists."

Today, in 2012, there are still millions of deaths from tuberculosis worldwide. Yet, if there existed a simple cure such as the one above, why is TB still a serious illness around the world?

The reason that the remedy above was not made available "from all chemists" is that commercially sold juices would require to be heated for storage reasons in order to be made available on the shelves – and that would be enough to destroy the life-giving and healing enzymes in these juices.

But another factor that should be remembered is that raw juices would bring no profits to the massive drug industry – it would only benefit the greengrocer. And, besides, it would take the care of health conditions out of the hands of the medical fraternity and place it in the hands of the sufferers themselves, putting, perhaps, doctors – and the drug industry – out of business.

There is an astonishing gap in the training of our doctors. There is virtually no instruction at all in the relationship between human diet and health, despite evidence from all over the world during the last 150 years or so – anecdotal as well as scientific.

Although the recent Channel 4 television programme, *The Food Hospital*, introduced the subject to the British public for the first time, it only scratched the surface of the far bigger story.

This book contains compelling evidence to show much more – that almost certainly your chronic health condition, whatever it is – whether mental or physical – can respond favourably to a mere change of diet. However, as there is no profit in diet for the drug industry, this approach is not encouraged, and, indeed, most decidedly discouraged. Remember, your well-meaning doctor can only use treatments that he has been taught at medical school. And using natural foods is not one of them.

Can the drug industry be that powerful, that it can dictate what treatment you get, choosing those that benefit them financially over harmless natural diet approaches? Dr James Howenstine M.D. states that the pharmaceutical industry has gained almost total control over the curricula taught in medical schools.[1] Even articles published in medical journals are influenced by the drug industry. Their control extends to deciding who receives research grants and what the recipients are allowed to study with these grants.

This control over research expenditures prevents research that might lead to cures for serious diseases such as cancer, schizophrenia, HIV, or Alzheimer's Disease. In America, Dr Howenstine observes, the pharmaceutical industry has established the precedent with the state boards of medical licence that any therapies that do not use pharmaceutical drugs (such as dietary approaches) are quackery which is dangerous to the public and should be suppressed.

The pressure for doctors to prescribe drug treatment, and drug treatment only, has caused great personal anguish and financial loss to many innovative physicians who have dared to treat patients with dietary approaches that can indeed produce cures. Often these doctors – mostly in the USA – must spend large amounts of money defending themselves from attempts to remove their licences.

Dr Herbert Shelton, a famous physiologist who ran a highly successful health clinic using fasting and diet in San Antonio, Texas, stated that with chronic health conditions, drugs fail to cure 98% of the time – a little known fact amongst the general public, who are inundated with daily newspaper reports reporting the latest "progress" in medical science towards a cure for this or that illness. With chronic illnesses such as arthritis, drug treatment may help for an hour or two, but after their effect wears off the patient will still have arthritis. There has been no actual cure. So it is with the vast majority of long-standing health complaints treated with medication.

THE MISSING PIECE OF THE JIGSAW

Can the mere act of cooking our food be behind the soaring illness statistics in our modern society? Even though we have been cooking food for thousands of years, could we still be badly getting it wrong? Everything points to it. And I will present that evidence throughout this book.

Can a raw or nearly-raw diet really bring about recovery from long-standing, stubborn illnesses, both mental and physical? Can illnesses that doctors cannot presently cure really be cured by eating as primitive man did, bearing in mind that cancers and other common illnesses were unknown in these earlier times? Could the cause of your long-term, perhaps life-long, condition be as simple as the food on your plate that you eat day in, day out? Because our medical scientists refuse to even consider our diet as a likely candidate for the cause of most chronic diseases, is this the reason that they are missing the most powerful influence on our health that exists?

There have been many studies over the last 100 years – in animal and man – showing how illness can come about as a consequence of eating the wrong food, and, importantly, showing how illness can be reversed if the wrong diet is removed and replaced with the correct one.

This book is filled with the evidence, gathered from medical research and studies from world-famous universities and colleges, medical institutions, clinics and hospitals, from all around the world.

There is an old saying that you can stumble over the truth, pick yourself up, and simply walk on as if nothing happened. By reading this book, you are right now stumbling over the truth – do not walk away without learning from it.

People in primitive societies who ate food as it was intended to be eaten – pristine, pure – and grown on soil, free from chemicals, had superb health and suffered no illness. Certainly cancer and a host of common complaints, including mental illness, rampant as they are today, were unknown in such societies.

One famous doctor, Sir Robert McCarrison, who was Director of Nutrition in India in the 1930s, came across a remote society called the Hunzas, who were cut off from outside influences by their very remoteness. There were no roads in and out of their villages. McCarrison observed that they had great strength and endurance, as well as perfect skin, superb physiques, beautiful teeth and extremely warm personalities. They would work in their fields until they were well into their 90s – middle-aged by their standards. They were also completely free from disease (as wild animals are) and lived to an advanced age. Their food was grown on pristine, natural soil. Their water came from glaciers in the mountains.

McCarrison gradually worked out that the reason for their superb health and freedom from illness was their completely natural diet. He was later to experiment with white rats, and, later, monkeys, to see if he could produce illness in these animals by feeding them cooked foods. He did, and you will learn more of this later.

Dr Francis Pottenger carried out the famous Pottenger Cats studies, whereby he divided 900 cats into two groups, feeding one group a completely raw diet, and the other a cooked diet. He was not only able to produce great health in the raw group, free from disease, but he produced dozens of ailments – mental as well as physical – in the cats that were fed cooked foods. Furthermore, Pottenger was able to **reverse** these illnesses by returning the ill animals to a raw diet. Again, you will read more of this later.

Every living organism in the world eats its food raw; all animals eat raw, all fish, all insects, all birds eat raw. They may die of injury or by being attacked by other animals, but disease as we know it in our human, cooked-food society, simply does not occur in the wild.

Illness in wild nature is virtually non-existent. You will read evidence of this later. Animals that are domesticated, or kept in zoos, generally do not have access to completely natural diets, and often eat cooked foods. Consequently, these animals are not as healthy as those in the wild. You may hear that animals in zoos live longer in captivity than in the wild. However, that is the reverse of the truth.

Man is the only animal that cooks his food. And man is the only animal to suffer from health conditions that, instead of improving because of the so-called progress in medical science, are becoming more and more numerous.

In America, where matters of health generally will spread to the UK sooner or later, there are 125 million people who suffer from a chronic complaint. That is predicted to rise to 171m by 2020, a matter of a few years.[2] How can this be, when we hear all the time about the "great progress" being made in medicine?

You will learn in this book that such "great progress" is very far from what is reality, and instead – contrary to what we are all led to believe – medical science cannot cure (and I mean *cure*) the vast majority of illnesses. You will learn that our doctors, well-meaning and dedicated professionals that they are, are simply given no training in the connection between the food that we eat and the many health conditions that have been shown to be brought on by a cooked, unnatural diet – for cooking is unnatural.

Within these pages you will be shown the evidence that highlights the vast difference in health that can be attained if you choose to eat, if not a fully raw diet, then a part-raw diet – organic preferably.

You may think that to eat this way would be unworkable, impractical, in our busy modern lives. But if you have a chronic, debilitating illness, you should welcome a means of recovery that doesn't involve toxic drugs, but merely a change of food.

Your diet does not have to be all raw, but a faster recovery will occur if it is. You can still recover from illness by using part-raw. Remember too, that whilst many people will think "Oh, rabbit food – I could never live on THAT!", primitive societies ate their entire diet that way and were completely free from disease – and happy! So how could *they* be happy on such a "rabbit-food" diet? Simple – they have not had their palate, or taste, distorted by long-term usage of cooked and junk foods. Their palates were normal, and they relished raw foods. Your palate – believe it or not – will change so that you too can relish eating a great variety of raw foods.

It will not be as hard as you think.

I recall, when visiting a Natural Hygiene clinic in Florida many years ago, how Dr Frank Sabatino, who was in charge there, would give his daily lecture to all the new patients, advising them on changing their diet to a more natural one. He said that when people first came, they would always complain about the diet they were given, which was comprised mostly of raw salads. But after a couple of weeks they would report that "the chef has greatly improved – the food tastes lovely now".

Of course, the chef hadn't changed, and the food itself hadn't changed; it was their *palates* that had normalised! They were now experiencing food in a way that had been lost to them for decades, probably for the first time in their entire lives.

When man was first put on Earth, he had no cooker, no stove, and, until he discovered fire, there was none. He would have used his instinct to choose his food in the form of foliage from bushes and trees; fruits, berries, vegetables, nuts and plants; and occasionally animals and fish – if he were near water. And, of course, his diet was completely raw, even eating the fish in its natural state (you will learn later of isolated societies, completely free from disease, which also ate their fish raw).

Cooking food destroys the life-giving enzymes that come within natural foods. Enzymes are responsible for thousands of different biochemical actions within the body and are destroyed at temperatures above 118 degrees F. The pasteurisation (heating) of milk, alone, for example, occurs by the application of heat upwards of 161 degrees F.

It must also be remembered that all chemical functions in the body, both for normal metabolism and for detoxification, are entirely dependent on enzymes. The more work to be done, the more enzymes are required. To make enzymes, the body needs colloidal minerals of all kinds, the best source of which, by far, are fresh, raw fruit and vegetables.[3]

Virtually all processed foods – tinned, packaged, bottled, etc – have been heated in the process of becoming shelf-ready – and are therefore deficient in enzymes.

Enzymes are the catalysts manufactured by the living cells of plant or animal tissue to carry out the chemical processes which allow the cells to continue their existence as a living force.

When the enzymes within a seed are destroyed, the seed has lost its potency for growth and is described as being dead. Whether a food can be declared "alive" or "dead" is dependent upon whether the enzymes are alive or have been destroyed by the heat-sensitive enzymes.

Early man, by eating a raw diet, had robust health and lived long, fruitful lives – quite the contrary to what you hear spouted by those who simply do not know the truth or, indeed, have vested interests in keeping you misinformed.

Our family doctors are honest, hard-working professionals, and indeed well meaning, but they cannot know what they are not taught. And they are not taught at medical school that human diet, if cooked, can result over decades in ill health, and they are not taught that, by reversing that practice – by eliminating cooking and eating raw – health disorders can be *reversed*.

Furthermore, they are not taught that the diet of the parents can have an enormous influence on the health of the offspring, and, notwithstanding, any illness passed down from the parents can still be overcome through dietary means. You will learn that later in the section on the Gerson therapy, and also in the Pottenger Cats study, where the same process applies to animals.

Medical science today still struggles to come up with drugs that can cure TB, which is now, in 2012, on the rise again in Western society.

Remember, too, that, whilst we take doctors and hospitals for granted – after all, we have grown up with them – doctors and hospitals are *unnatural*! There were no such things thousands of years ago. Doctors and hospitals are modern "inventions", after all. When we were placed on Earth, no such entities existed originally. We were designed to heal our own bodies. And that innate ability still exists within all of us; we are self-healing organisms. We are all capable of healing our bodies, if not damaged irreparably by injury, that is, and the extent to which we can recover our health is dependent upon the nutrition that we feed into our bodies.

Returning to the TB cure above, despite TB being on the increase, doctors and hospitals still do not employ nutrition as a means of recovery for their patients, despite growing evidence that such a change in lifestyle can afford the patient great improvement in health.

The importance of enzymes in our food cannot be over-stated. We know heating destroys these catalysts required for many biochemical reactions, but many other changes can occur in the body as a consequence of the simple cooking of our foods.

The "anti-stiffness" chemical of raw cream, discovered by Wulzen and Wagtendonk of Oregon State University, is known to be destroyed by boiling or pasteurisation.[4] The "filtrate-factor" of certain vegetables, which controls the ageing process of the body, is reported by Morgan and Simms to be easily lost when vegetables are boiled. Certain hormones, including those from the adrenal cortex, are also heat-sensitive and destroyed in the process of heating – pasteurising – milk.

Many other changes in the body occur when consuming cooked foods; some known, some yet to be discovered.

But evidence of the unnaturalness of cooking our foods is shown in the fact that leukocytosis, an increase in the number of white blood cells, follows the exclusive consumption of cooked foods.

In medicine, an increase in the number of white blood cells, together with disturbances in the percentages of different kinds of white cells, is known to indicate that some kind of disease process is going on in our body. In time of infectious illness, or when harmful extraneous substances are introduced into our system, these changes in white blood cell development always take place. We have reason to believe, therefore, that the leukocytosis following the consumption of cooked food is an indicator that our body is telling us that we are indeed doing something wrong.

Biologists have sometimes referred to it as "digestive leukocytosis" and, unaware of the difference between eating cooked food or raw food, consider it a normal reaction to the digestive process.

However, Dr. Paul Kouchakoff, of the Institute of Clinical Chemistry in Lausanne, Switzerland – a Nobel Prize winner – conducted some 300 detailed experiments which indicated that leukocytosis was the specific effect of eating heat-processed foods and that it never occurred after a meal of raw food![5]

Reporting at the First International Congress of Microbiology at Paris in 1930, Dr. Kouchakoff pointed out that temporary leukocytosis followed the consumption of foods heated to about 83-87 degrees C (181-188 degrees F). If certain types of raw food were added to the cooked meal, leukocytosis would be prevented, though when foods were heated above 100 degrees C (212 degrees F), no amount of raw foods would prevent the condition. Likewise, when heat-processed foods which had also been subjected to complex manufacturing processes were consumed, leukocytosis was unavoidable.

This book is about how many long-term illnesses can be removed from the body by the simple expedient of eating foods that are enzyme-rich and, therefore, raw.

So, why is this not known by medical science, the practitioners of which could simply apply this diet to their patients and restore us to health?

Because the only people who would benefit, as has been said previously, would be the greengrocers. The global pharmaceutical giants ("Big Pharma") would see their profits seriously affected, and, in common with any industry that is threatened, they will do anything they can to ensure they retain their vast profits.

The fact that money can even be a factor in your illness at all should be *unthinkable*. But you will learn later in this book that the huge profits in drugs play a big part in the treatment of illness nowadays.

And if you think that medical science would be whiter than white, and that no such thing as mere money can get in the way of curing, then prepare to have your eyes opened.

Amongst many, many others who have uncovered fraud, bribery and corruption within the drug industry, Gwen Olsen, a pharmaceutical industry insider for more than ten years, uncovered "staggering" fraud and misrepresentation in that industry, which she exposed in her 2009 book, *Confessions of an Rx Drug Pusher*.[6]

Despite most of us being led to believe that our health is in good hands, medical research has no cure for arthritis, cancer, heart disease, mental illness, and the whole gamut of chronic conditions that besets mankind in the 21st century.

The normal treatment for most conditions may be drugs, but they are only of temporary assistance. They are not *cures*.

You may take medication for your arthritis, which may help alleviate the condition for an hour or so, but once the effect of the medication wears off, you will still have your arthritis. There has been no *cure*.

Similarly, cutting off a cancerous breast is hardly a *cure* for breast cancer. It is little different to cutting off someone's head because he has a headache ...

There is no question about it – our health is getting worse. Never in the history of mankind has there been such a sick generation as we are today. The number of maladies, of all kinds, is escalating dramatically. Our health is getting worse – far worse – than ever before. More people are developing chronic conditions, mental illness, cancers, and other degenerative diseases, now, in this 21st century, than ever before in the entire history of the planet.

Drugs may have their place – but are not necessary – in sorting out the occasional headache or upset tummy. These are acute conditions which are self-limiting, which means that they will go away of their own accord anyway. Any drug given will simply paralyse the pain at the site of the disorder whilst the body gets to work carrying out the repair.

However, for the really debilitating conditions – the depressions, the psoriases, the cancers, the arthritises – drugs simply do not produce a cure.

Dr Herbert Shelton used to say that, before you can cure a disease, you have first to find the *cause* of the disease and then remove that cause.

Our existing medical paradigm does not cater for that approach.

In fact, Dr Shelton estimated that medicine cannot cure 98% of all diseases. He considered it was 100%, but he left room for those who would argue the point!

This little-known statistic will certainly take the average reader by surprise. But if you think about it, all the treatments available are only symptomatic and not curative.

Doctors can practise only what they have been taught at medical school.

And what they are taught is to dispense drugs, drugs, and more drugs. Little or no thought is given to finding an actual cure.

And certainly little or no training is given in *natural* nutrition and the disorders that can appear as a consequence of violating natural laws.

You will find, throughout this book, real evidence that a raw, or even part-raw, diet can restore health, removing conditions that have baffled doctors and medical research for hundreds of years.

Whilst this book will give new hope to people with "incurable" conditions, whether physical or mental, it must be made clear that if you are on any medication at all, it is essential that you consult with your doctor first about the possibility of coming off, or reducing them gradually, as stopping drug treatment can be dangerous and it needs monitoring, preferably by the doctor who prescribed them.

2.

Some Examples of Raw Food Cures

Many examples are given throughout this book of recovery from disease by the use of raw foods.

Evidence of the importance of raw food in healing was found at the Olive View Sanatorium in the county of Los Angeles in the 1950s.

Dr H. E. Kirschner was placed in charge of 200 tuberculosis patients in his clinic. Some of the patients had spent as long as nine years on their backs with very little progress towards recovery. The diet was composed largely of spaghetti, macaroni, and other cooked foods.

Dr Kirschner added a glass of green drink, consisting of the raw juices of alfalfa, spinach, and parsley, to the diet of each of these patients every day.

Results were very favourable, and the course of the patients was changed to recovery. Some of the patients who had been considered hopeless were able to get out of bed within six to eight months.

This may seem a long time, but remember that they were still indulging in their old cooked diet at the same time – remarkable proof of the healing power of raw juices/foods.

That also presents the evidence that you do not have to consume an entirely raw diet to make recovery; however, the more raw in your diet, the quicker recovery will be achieved.

In Dr Kirschner's private practice, raw carrot juice, in addition to the green juice mixture, was included in the diet of tubercular patients, which brought about more rapid recovery than did the green juice alone.

Dr Kirschner also reported that other chronic ailments can be treated very successfully with raw vegetable juices, taken in some cases in amounts exceeding two quarts per day.

He reported recoveries from heart disease, prostate gland disease, cancer, neuritis, and haemorrhoids, through the use of raw juices.

In one diabetic case, remarkable improvement was noted within the first 21 days of treatment, and the insulin dosage was reduced from 15 to 5 units per day.

The most remarkable case history cited by Dr Kirschner, however, was that of a severe case of splenic leukaemia. The patient in this instance was given raw carrot juice – small quantities at first, with gradual increases to very large quantities – and her weight increased from 65 lbs to 135 lbs. Recovery was complete within 18 months, and at no later time was there any recurrence of the disease.

Another fabulous example of how diet can restore health to tuberculosis patients, without drugs of any kinds, is given in the chapter about The Gerson Therapy.

The value of raw liver in treating pernicious anaemia has also been known for almost 100 years.

Drs Murphy and Minot were curing severe cases of this disease with raw liver back in the 1920s.

They claimed there was some unidentifiable factor in the food which stimulated the growth of red blood cells. At first, this was called the "red blood vitamin". It is now known that there are two such factors, folic acid and vitamin B12, both of which are destroyed by heat!

Therefore, whereas cooked liver is virtually useless in these cases, raw liver brings about consistent and rapid recovery. For perhaps the same reason, raw liver, given to weak and undersized children, has been reported to increase vigour and strength and improve their rate of growth.

Other European physicians using raw beef juices (blood, essentially) for tuberculosis had similar success at that time. Prof Charles Richet was among the first to use raw beef juice in the treatment of tuberculosis, and he reported excellent results in this practice. Later, other physicians followed the same method, applying the term "Zomotherapy" to designate treatment of disease with raw meat or raw meat juice. They claimed success with zomotherapy in treating many conditions, including anaemia, neurasthenia (now generally referred to as neurosis), debility, and latent, incipient, or active tuberculosis.

In Europe, a diet composed primarily of raw foods was employed in the treatment of disease as early as the latter part of the 19th century. At that time, the "Jungborn", a health resort located in the Hartz mountain region between Isenburg and Hartzburg, in Germany, was opened. The director of this institution was Adolph Just, a philosopher and naturalist, who concluded from his observations of wild and domestic animal life that only raw foods were capable of building the health, strength, and vigour that are normal in nature.

At his clinic, Mr Just provided sun and air baths, special water baths, and earth compresses as treatment, in addition to raw foods. The diet consisted in the main of fruits, berries, nuts, and milk in the uncooked state (unpasteurised, raw).

In 1896, Mr Just issued a number of case history records illustrating the results of his raw food and natural treatment therapy. Among the diseases reported cured or reduced were inflammatory rheumatism, consumption of the spinal cord, tuberculosis of the bones, dropsy, incipient dropsy, fistula of the rectum, cancer, nervous spasms, deafness, and various digestive ailments and sexual disorders.

Recoveries were often rapid as well as complete. Recovery from severe nervous disorders was achieved in ten weeks, from deafness in eight weeks, from inflammatory rheumatism in nine days, and from incipient dropsy in less than a week.

Great improvement in cases of different forms of consumption was noted during the first two weeks of treatment. The general success was attributed largely to the use of raw foods.

RAW MILK AND TUBERCULOSIS

An interesting example of this is afforded by a letter printed and signed by eight members of Parliament in England in the 1930s, in which important statistics on this question are referred to.

The letter stated:

"May we here adduce certain facts relating to a single county as recorded in the last report of the Medical Officer of Health for Hertfordshire: This county has a population of 420,000, and all the milk drunk by them is produced in the county.

During 1932 there were 45 deaths in all from surgical tuberculosis, of which 33 were children under 15. In 13 rural districts, where the whole supply is in the hands of small retailers of raw milk, there were no deaths at all during the year from surgical tuberculosis.

The highest death rate was in an urban area where the population lives under model conditions and practically all the milk supply is pasteurised."

A further study of the relationship between milk and tuberculosis was made by Dr MacDonald, Medical Officer to Dr Barnardo's Homes in England. Dr MacDonald reported that, among 750 children who were given pasteurised milk, along with other food for a period of five years, 14 cases of tuberculosis developed. Another 750 boys were given raw milk for an equal period of time, with the other conditions, including the rest of the diet being the same as with the other group. During this time, only one case of tuberculosis developed, which represents a 1,400 percent advantage for the unpasteurised group. It was also reported that chilblains were absent among the boys of this group, whereas they were quite common among those receiving pasteurised milk.

3.

Curing by Raw Foods

Over the past 100 or so years there have been many studies and reports showing how raw diets can improve or cure the health of patients with long-standing complaints.

Multiple sclerosis is deemed incurable by modern medicine.

But the experience of Dr Joseph Evers, in Germany, is important in this disease. He treated 600 cases of multiple sclerosis with diets containing no refined foods, and consisting chiefly of raw fruits, raw nuts, raw vegetable roots, raw honey, raw grain sprouts, uncooked coarse-rolled oats, wholemeal bread, raw ham, raw bacon, and raw chopped beef.

His dietary treatment was set up under the controls of recognised scientists and tested in different universities, clinics, hospitals, and sanatoriums. The results were surprisingly good and 42 percent of all patients showed improvement or complete recovery. This percentage may seem low, but for multiple sclerosis, which consistently fails to yield to orthodox medical treatment, a single recovery is worthy of note.

If the simple addition of certain raw foods to a normal diet produces startling changes in human health, it may be expected that a diet composed entirely, or nearly so, of raw foods would be much more beneficial and achieve more rapid and far-reaching results. This has been shown to be true at the Pottenger Sanatorium in California, where a large variety of raw foods has been employed for therapeutic purposes.

Dr Pottenger writes that "the highest grade of raw milk, raw meat, raw vegetables, and fruit products obtained" are used in the clinical work. He points out that "we have been able to improve the physiologic response of children who have previously been developing in a deficient manner, similar to the experimental animals which were fed upon heat-processed foods.

Even defective facial growth has been improved, and Pottenger states that "when additional growth stimulation is applied to certain deficient children at the right time, before they have attained facial growth, material changes in the contour of the face can be brought about without the application of surgical appliances."

During the year 1897, a famous healing institution was opened in Switzerland. This was the great Bircher-Benner clinic and sanatorium in Zurich.

Here extensive use has been made or raw foods, and some patients have been placed on an exclusive raw diet for a limited period of time when this was deemed necessary.

The late founder of the institution, Dr Bircher-Benner, stated that "raw vegetable food is the most potent healing factor that exists", which is able "to bring healing to very many widely spread disorders of health and serious diseases, in quite astonishing fashion, where all other curative measures have failed".[7]

He called raw food "sunlight food" and referred to his delicious preparations of fruits, vegetables, nuts, honey, milk, and other foods, all in their raw state, as "sunlight dishes".

The success of this sanatorium was so phenomenal that it attracted patients from all over the world. It was best known for its treatment of digestive diseases.

So astonishing was the recovery, on a strictly raw diet, of one supposedly incurable patient suffering from Herter-Heubner disease (also referred to as coeliac disease), that it attracted the attention of the children's hospital in Zurich, which in turn introduced a raw diet for its coeliac patients. The medical director of the hospital at the time published a monograph giving an account of the "staggering success" thus achieved.

Today, the Bircher-Benner clinics are still open in Europe, in Germany and Spain. They carry on the important work of their founder with equally satisfactory results.

Dr Bircher-Benner described raw food in relation to the "five zones of its influence". In the first zone, the effects are noticeable within a few days, with the "return of appetite, rapid fading of unnatural thirst" and "much better digestion".

In the second zone, embracing weeks of time, the circulatory system responds to the curative effects of raw food.

The third zone "needs months to become effective", though some improvement may be noticed almost immediately. It covers the endocrine glands and metabolism.

The fourth zone, embracing the capillary system and secondary effects on all parts of the organism, is reported by Dr Bircher-Benner as requiring one to three years, sometimes less, "to show the effects of its domain".

The entire four-fold action, according to Dr Bircher-Benner, "generally brings about a complete change in obstinate cases of many chronic conditions such as stomatitis and ulcers, sprue, amoebic dysentery, lambliasis and malaria, kidney troubles, jaundice, eczemas and urticaria, headaches, and schizophrenia, also in various cases of varicose, thrombophlebitis, and many other conditions".

The fifth zone applies to the constitution itself, from which our diseases and infections originate. It means a fundamental change in the physiological efficiency of the entire body, with new vitality and vigorous health.

At the First Medical Clinic of the University of Vienna, two scientists, Eppinger and Kaunitz, tested the Bircher-Benner raw food diets as a means of improving the interchange of energies and substances between the ends of the blood vessels (capillaries) and the tissue cells of the body.

Under normal conditions of life, the blood gives up its nutritive substances and the cells give up their waste substances in this interchange through two fine membranes and a narrow dividing interstice.

Often, however, the cells lose a part of their "selective capacity" because of salt penetrating the cell wall, distortion and spasms of the capillaries, a sticky coating of blood globules, waste products being scattered around the cells, and reduction of the chemical, physical, and electrical tensions which promote the nutritive interchange.

When this happens, cells cannot rejuvenate fast enough; bacteria tend to multiply too rapidly, and the general cause of many clinical symptoms of disease is in existence.

Eppinger and Kaunitz studied this condition and tried every possible means of restoring normal selective power in the cells once this had been lost.

Only one measure was found to be successful. This was the application of an exclusive raw food diet, "exactly according to the prescriptions of Dr Bircher-Benner". Under the influence of this diet, the life-giving tensions between capillaries and cells grew and the capillaries were slowly restored to a normal, vigorous condition.

In Munich, the German physicians, Friedrich and Peters, employed a raw diet consisting chiefly of fruits and vegetables, and small amounts of meat. Many severe cases of liver cirrhosis, with ascites, were treated.

Results, surprisingly, were quite successful, and a number of most striking cases have been cited by the physicians to show the value of raw foods in the treatment of this disease.[8]

Other physicians and scientists who have studied the raw diet in relation to therapeutic uses are D. C. Hare, J. F. Kinderheilk, W. Heupe, I. Kanai, and M. Kuratsune. Dr Hare, of the Royal Free Hospital in England, placed arthritic patients on an exclusive raw diet for two weeks, followed by a predominantly raw diet for several weeks. Most of the patients began to feel better within one to four weeks, with marked improvement continuing thereafter.

Kinderheilk found the raw diet to be of value in avitaminosis, nephritis, diabetes, and chronic constipation. In cases of cardiac disease, he noted that it promoted the excretion of superfluous water and was thus helpful to the patients.

Dr Heupe, working at the University Medical Polyclinic in Frankfurt, reported that the diet was an aid in the treatment of diarrhoea of children, in heart and kidney diseases, and in obesity and diabetes.

Kanai, of the University of Berlin, studied the effect of raw and cooked vegetarian diets on the oxidation of the body. He noted that oxidation was impaired by cooked vegetarian foods.

On the raw diet, the urinary output of nitrogen was greater, indicating better absorption, and the weight increase was better.[9]

Dr Kuratsune, of Kyushu University, Japan, also tested raw and cooked vegetarian diets, and reported results were decidedly better on the raw regime. Heated vegetables tended to produce anaemia, which was cured when raw vegetables were eaten.

Other diseases which had failed to yield to conventional medical care responded favourably to the raw diet.

In the UK, in the first half of the 20th century, doctors have been equally successful in utilising freshly-extracted raw juices for therapeutic purposes.

The Ministry of Health and Public Health Service Laboratory issued a report pointing out the value of using the juices of cabbage, kale, parsley, and other uncooked vegetables in the treatment of a wide variety of diseased conditions.

The report stated: "Juices are valuable in relief of hypertension, cardiovascular and kidney diseases and obesity. Good results have also been obtained in rheumatic, degenerative and toxic states. Juices have an all-round protective action. Good results can be obtained in treatment of peptic ulceration, also in treatment of chronic diarrhoea, colitis and toxaemia of gastro and intestinal origin."

The dental scientist, Dr Harold F. Hawkins, has reported that correct dietary control, with at least half of all foods used in their raw state, is of much more value in treating the symptoms of pyorrhea, including infection of the alveolar bone, which supports the teeth and gums.

According to Dr Hawkins, in caring for the pyorrhea patient, it is "essential" to work out a plan of eating that will include food that can be eaten raw, such as raw milk, raw eggs, oysters on the half shell, raw vegetable salads, and raw fruit.

Dr Hawkins states that, when an adequate diet is followed, "the gum tone usually shows a definite improvement in 60 to 90 days, and the X-rays show an improvement in bone density in about a year."[10]

During the years 1929, 1930, and 1931, Dr Milton T. Hanke, working through the facilities provided by the University of Chicago and the Chicago Dental Research Club, studied hundreds of school children in the city of Mooseheart, Illinois, to determine the effects of adding the raw juices of citrus fruits to a conventional diet.[11]

During the first year, the children were studied as controls; the second year was the test period, and the third was the recheck period.

Approximately 16 ounces of freshly extracted raw orange juice, plus the raw juice of one lemon, were added to the diet of each of 341 children on each day of the test period.

This brought about a sharp increase in growth rate over the control period, as well as a 50 percent reduction in the incidence of dental caries and the almost complete disappearance of gingivitis.

During the recheck period, when the quantity of juice was reduced to three ounces a day, the accelerated growth was maintained, though dental decay again increased and most of the gingivitis reappeared.

Other fruits and juices also have therapeutic qualities. The "grape cure" is well known in parts of Europe and has found extensive employment in the sanatoriums and resorts of Merano, Italy, parts of France, and southern Germany.

The patients of these institutions were fed almost exclusively on raw grapes for four to six weeks at a time, starting with about a pound a day and gradually increasing the amount to five to eight pounds a day.

Johanna Brandt, author of *The Grape Cure*, reported a number of cures from cancer through the employment of the raw grape diet, and others have used it successfully in the treatment of constipation, rheumatism, catarrh, gallstones, eczema, jaundice, malaria, haemorrhages, and other ailments.

Grape cures are even recommended in certain mental disturbances and in weakened conditions of the entire muscular system, including the heart.

Basil Shackleton used the grape cure to cure himself of an abscess in his one kidney, after having one removed because of illness, also wrote a book, similarly entitled *The Grape Cure*.

Raw cabbage juice has been used with remarkable success in treating ulcers. Dr Garnett Chaney, at Stanford University, treated 63 ulcer patients with one quart of raw cabbage juice per day, and 60 of these showed pronounced healing.[12]

In most cases, the pain disappeared within a few days and recovery was complete within three weeks or less.

Six patients with "huge" ulcers required 56 days of treatment. The three patients who failed to respond had dense scar tissue in the stomach and liver damage before treatment started.

Dr Chaney's experience was almost duplicated by Dr William Shive and his colleagues at the University of Texas. Dr Shive found that raw cabbage juice – as well as the juices of some other vegetables – tends to prevent ulcers and to cure them.

He studied 100 cases in which the ulcerous condition was so severe that the use of the bland diet and anti-ulcer drugs had failed.

But the drinking of one quart of fresh, raw cabbage juice per day by these patients brought about marked beneficial results.

The use of raw cabbage juice in amounts less than one quart per day promotes less rapid recovery than does the full quota, but it is of definite value, and even a glass of juice per day tends to reduce or eliminate the pain in some cases.

The raw cabbage juice is also an important aid to normal elimination and it improves the general health of the ulcer patient, as well as promoting recovery of his primary affliction.

The "scraped raw apple" diet is an old German remedy for both diarrhoea and constipation. Modern scientists have employed raw apple in the treatment of these same conditions with very good effects.

T. L. Birnberg treated diarrhoea in children with raw, grated apple and obtained completely successful results in 88 percent of all cases. He noted relief from abdominal pain was achieved almost immediately, normal stools were achieved in 24 hours, reduction in fever within 48 hours, and disappearance of mucous in 60 hours.

The beneficial effects of raw apple in these cases are attributed to the presence of "hydrophilic colloids" in the food which absorb excessive water and furnish bulk to control peristalsis.[13]

It was concluded from a 1990 German study of raw food that it is "an integral component of human nutrition, and is a necessary precondition for an intact immune system. Its therapeutic effect is complex, and a variety of influences of raw food and its constituents on the immune system have been documented. Such effects include antibiotic, antiallergic, tumour-protective, immunomodulatory, and anti-inflammatory actions. In view of this, uncooked food can be seen as a useful adjunct to drugs in the treatment of allergic, rheumatic and infectious diseases."[14]

In 1998, in Finland, a number of studies using raw food on rheumatoid arthritis patients showed that the diet reduced pain, improved their sleep and greatly improved joint stiffness. The researchers found that the reduction of their pain, swelling of joints and morning stiffness, all got worse after returning to a cooked diet. They also concluded that: "It appears that the raw food approach leads to a lessening of several health risk factors to cardiovascular diseases and cancer".[15]

In the 1950s, in Denmark, an exclusive raw diet consisting of fruits, vegetables, nuts, cornmeal, sprouted grains and legumes, honey and milk was given to all patients who visited the "Humlegaarden", a sanatorium located near Humlebek.

Dr Kristine Nolfi, medical director of the sanatorium, was formerly associated in medicine and surgery with the Communal Hospital in Copenhagen and also in Paediatrics at the State Hospital.

During her years of hospital training, she suffered from weak digestion and catarrh of the stomach, and in the winter of 1940 and 1941 she observed the symptoms of cancer. A trial microscopy taken at the Radium Centre in Copenhagen was positive, indicating there were cancer cells.

Dr Nolfi treated herself with an exclusive raw diet and recovered excellent health (see her fuller account later).

This success prompted her to open the "Humlegaarden", where not only the patients, but even members of the hospital staff, lived entirely upon foods which had not been treated by heating.

About one thousand patients annually visited this clinic, and doctors from Denmark and other countries also visited the place and made observations which were utilised in their practices.

The therapeutic successes attained at the Humlegaarden are said to be phenomenal. Dr Nolfi attributed this to the consumption of raw foods, and in particular to the use of raw garlic and raw potatoes. Patients at this clinic recovered from all manner of diseases, including cancer, sterility, obesity, diabetes, heart debilitation, high blood pressure, rheumatism, epilepsy, asthma, and many other conditions. In some cases, even grey hair darkened in colour.

According to Dr Nolfi, the raw diet "has a curative effect not only for a particular disease and on an individual organ, but on the organism as a whole. It cures not only the diseases contracted during our short lifespan, but also those determined by hereditary predisposition."

You have to be aware that, when a raw diet is taken, the diet does not specifically target just one illness. If you have several conditions, it will restore health to the entire body, which will, therefore, mean that all conditions can be rectified by the one dietary approach.

This is not that difficult to understand when you consider that the nutrients in the diet enter the bloodstream, and the blood reaches every part of the body. If there are blockages – anywhere in the system – that could be responsible for symptoms beyond that blockage, then the slowly clearing away of such plaque in the blood vessels will occur, if the diet is maintained long enough in order to achieve this work.

Sadly, we understand that, although the Humlegaarden still exists, it has been taken over by orthodox medical practitioners, not conversant with the dietary approach.

The need for a complete overhaul of the food that we eat is evidenced by the increasing number of people suffering from long-standing illness in both the UK and America, as well as most other countries who eat in a similar fashion.

Instead of medical science – which we blindly believe can solve all our health problems – providing cures, it appears itself to be *part* of the problem by accepting the *status quo* and not looking into the link between chronic illness and our food. They refuse to budge on the issue that diet is critical to our health and, instead, just spend billions on research for more and more drugs; none of which has provided the slightest cure for any disease.

Paradoxically, it is the *ignorance* of scientists, who are unwilling to look at a veritable mountain of "anecdotal" reports of people recovering from chronic illness, cancers, etc, from all over the world during the past century, in order to convert them into serious research, serious solutions to illness.

Their preference for money-spinning drugs which can never cure any illness brought about by bad diet is mind-boggling.

Instead of these reports being seriously looked at – along with a ton of clinical evidence from institutes around the world – they are discredited and dismissed by vested interests who put profit in front of health.

You only have to read reviews on books by authors who cured themselves of cancer, written by those who do not want it to be true, to realise there are dark forces at work, who have no interest in helping people recover from life-threatening illness, but who have every interest in protecting their own financial status.

Accusations of such reports being "pseudo-science" have been hurled at these accounts of recovery. But the truth is, if it is pseudo-science, it is achieving far, far better results than the so-called science that criticises them, when they themselves have absolutely *no* solution to illness themselves.

Partnership for Solutions, an initiative of Johns Hopkins University and The Robert Wood Johnson Foundation, collects health statistics and calculates future projections. They define "chronic illness" the following way:

"A chronic condition lasts a year or longer, limits what one can do and may require ongoing care. More than 125 million Americans have at least one chronic condition and 60 million have more than one condition. Examples of chronic conditions are diabetes, cancer, glaucoma and heart disease. The number of people with chronic conditions is growing at an alarming rate. In 2000, 20 million more people had one or more chronic conditions than the number originally estimated in 1996. By the year 2020, 25% of the American population will be living with multiple chronic conditions, and costs for managing these conditions will reach $1.07 trillion. … The number of people with chronic conditions is projected to increase from 125 million in 2000 to 171 million in the year 2030."[16]

4.

The Pottenger Cats Study

Perhaps the most important of all the animal experiments with raw and cooked foods are those of Dr Francis Pottenger, Jr, one of the world's great physicians and food scientists.

These were conducted at the long-established Pottenger Sanatorium in Monrovia, California, and covered a ten-year period. His famous book showing the results of his experiments is *Pottenger Cats: A Study in Nutrition.*[17]

Both white rats and cats were employed in the feeding studies. Rats given heated milk suffered from many kinds of deterioration, and the change in trabeculation of the bones was particularly noticeable.

With the cats, the experiments were reported in great detail and covered a large number of animals. A total of 900 cats were studied, and complete records were kept of nearly 600 of them.

Through generation after generation the animals were studied, and Dr Pottenger has issued the detailed results of the experiments as they apply to growth, reproduction, and all phases of the animals' health.

In these tests the animals were fed on meat scraps (including the muscle, bone and viscera), milk, and cod liver oil.

The animals were divided into various groups, depending on the condition, whether heated or unheated, in which their foods were given. Some of the cats were fed entirely on raw meat and raw milk; others were given two-thirds cooked meat and one-third raw milk. In some cases, raw meat and pasteurised milk were used.

A number of cats were also fed sweetened condensed milk, evaporated milk, or raw metabolised vitamin D milk with raw meat. Cod liver oil was used by all animal groups.

The cats fed entirely on raw meat and raw milk remained in excellent health in all cases. Physical development was virtually perfect and the cats reproduced in homogeneity from one generation to the next, maintaining large skulls and thoraxes, broad faces with prominent malar and orbital arches, broad and well-formed dental arches, adequate nasal cavities, and large and long bodies.

The cats were quite free from vermin, infections, and parasites. The membranes were firm and of good pink colour. All evidence of degeneration was absent.

Abortion occurred very seldom; the size of the average litter was five, and all of the mother cats nursed their young in a normal manner. The cats possessed excellent equilibrium. Organic development was complete and normal physical and mental function was the general rule. Death resulted only from old age or injuries sustained in fighting.

None of the cats died from disease.

Cats which were fed the cooked-meat scraps were defective in many respects. They were smaller in build and the bones were smaller in diameter. In some cases the bones would grow out of proportion, with the hind legs being much longer than the forelegs. The animals did not reproduce in homogeneity, each kitten being of a different skeletal pattern.

There were variations of facial structure similar to those of human beings. Configuration of the skulls was different in each individual cat. Often there would be marked failure in the development of the upper lip and in some cases a mandibular protrusion.

Dental conditions would usually remain fairly good in the first generation, though gingivitis occasionally developed. Second-generation animals usually had much smaller primary teeth than normal and there was irregular spacing of the teeth.

Bleeding of gums would increase considerably. Some teeth would be lost. In the third generation, loss of most of the teeth through decalcification and pyorrhea would be common.

Dental development was generally so irregular that the development of the whole face was interfered with.

There was severe impairment of bone composition in all cases. The calcium content would fall from the normal 12 to 18 percent of bone weight in healthy animals to 8 to 12 percent in the first generation; 3½ to 7 percent in the second generation; and finally 1½ to 3 percent in the third generation.

The phosphorous content also became progressively less, and by the third generation the bones would be very porous and similar to rubber. This resulted in bow legs, distorted spines, and other deformities.

Reproductive efficiency was greatly lowered. Abortion ran from 25 percent in the first generation to as high as 70 percent in the second generation. Deliveries were very difficult and many cats died in labour. Often the mother was unable to lactate.

The mortality rate of the kittens was very high, many of them even being too frail to nurse. In a number of cases the mother would steadily decline in health following birth of the kittens and die about three months later.

Others had increasing difficulty with subsequent pregnancies and some failed to become pregnant. In the males there was disturbance of genital development and descent of the testes. Sterility was so common that raw-food males had to be used for all breeding purposes.

Development of the secondary sexual characteristics was incomplete. The degree of masculinity and femininity was lessened and cats of both sexes tended to become more neutral in appearance. For instance, X-ray pictures showed that skulls of third-generation cooked-fed animals had neutral profiles for both sexes, as contrasted with the difference in raw-fed animals.

At the same time, sex interest was very slack; in many cases it was perverted, with some cats developing into true homosexuals.

Most of the cats fed cooked meat were very irritable and would occasionally viciously bite the keeper. Intestinal parasites and vermin were very common. Skin lesions and allergies became worse from one generation to the next.

Pneumonia and emphysema were the most common causes of death in the adult stock. A great number died from diarrhoea followed by pneumonia.

No cats fed the cooked diet survived the sixth month of life in the third generation. Among the diseased conditions that were found upon autopsy were: osteomyelitis, cardiac lesions, hyperopia, thyroid disease, hepatitis, nephritis, paralysis, meningitis, cystitis, arthritis, rickets, enlarged colon, bronchitis, fatty infiltration of the muscles, rachitic rosary of the ribs, and enlarged bladder.

Cats fed upon a combination of two-thirds pasteurised milk and one-third raw meat presented much the same deterioration as the other animals. Reproductive efficiency was lowered; skeletal structures were severely impaired; dental irregularity and gingivitis were common, and all kittens showed some form of deficiency in development.

Cats fed evaporated milk were damaged even more, and sweetened condensed milk produced the most marked deficiencies of all.

Even the raw metabolised vitamin D milk (from cattle fed irradiated yeast) proved harmful. The males showed osseous disturbances following its use, and the adult males died within 10 months, with the young males failing to live beyond even the second month.

In some instances, cats which had been fed either cooked meat or one of the forms of heated or vitamin D milk would be placed upon a completely raw diet, which would be continued in subsequent generations. Improvement in resistance to disease was noticed in the first and second generations in the "regenerating" animals, though there were still allergic manifestations, and reproduction was erratic.

In the third generation there was considerable further improvement, and by the fourth generation some of the animals returned to completely normal skeletal and tissue form.

From these experiments, as well as all others which have been reported, results of feeding raw and cooked foods under laboratory conditions become readily apparent. It follows that, almost without exception, experimental animals thrive well on an exclusive diet of raw foods.

With general uniformity, they immediately suffer from various forms of deterioration – physical, sexual, and mental – when given various forms of cooked foods. It has indeed been shown that members of certain animal species fail to reach maturity and reproduce if sufficient cooked foods are included in their diet.

The degree of damage may vary to some degree with different animals, but in no instance have large quantities of heat-processed foods been consumed over a long period of time without some harm being observed.

The contrast is clearly observed in all cases, and the many different animals used in the experiments show that the results do not apply to only certain kinds of experimental animals, but may be accepted as a general principle in all such nutritional work.

As for applying his results to human nutrition, Dr Pottenger said, "While no attempt will be made to correlate the changes in the animals studied with malformations found in humans, the similarity is so obvious that parallel pictures will suggest themselves."

It is a strange paradox that most of the criticism comes from advocates of the present system of medicine which employs drugs, not diet. And what do these drug researchers use in their research? Yes – animals!

There is no similar experiment in all of medical literature. The findings were supervised by Dr Pottenger, along with Dr Alvin Foord, professor of pathology at the University of Southern California and pathologist at the Huntington Memorial Hospital in Pasadena. These studies met the most rigorous scientific standards of their day.

5.

Man's Diet Should be Simple
– and Natural

Every animal in the wild has its own specific diet. The elk will eat grasses, leaves and shrubs. The tiger will eat deer, buffalo and other animals. The ape will eat leaves, shoots of plants, termites, and other insects.

Every animal has its specific range of diet. But no animal has the equivalent of man's vast selection of what is available to eat.

Man's diet is filled with so many artificial foods that one needs only to walk into a grocery store or a sweet or candy shop to see the mountainous bounty of packaged "foods": a million miles from the animal kingdom's equivalent. A further million miles from what man was intended to   eat.

Take any of the above animals away from their normal diet and give them the sort of "food" that we apparently consume without concern, and it won't be long before they fall ill.

Feed a dog on white bread alone and it would be dead in a matter of weeks.

You could not give a tiger herbs and grasses to eat without it becoming ill. You could equally not give an elk meat to eat without it suffering. You could not give any of these animals white bread, jam, processed cereals coated with refined sugar, pasteurised milk, and so on, without them being seriously affected.

The animal research throughout this book shows just what can happen when you feed animals food which they were not intended to eat in nature.

Dr Pottenger showed that if you gave white rats the food of specific Indian cultures, the rats would soon exhibit symptoms similar to those suffered by the Indians in that society.

All of the above animals – the elk, the tiger, the ape – all animals from the same genus, have diets that are quite limited, but they thrive and live healthy lives on such diets. And that is how they were meant to live.

So it is that the diet for one elephant will be the intended diet for all elephants. The diet for one mongoose will be the intended diet for all mongooses. The diet for one hummingbird will be the intended diet for all hummingbirds, and so on.

However, the one thing in common with all these animals, and, indeed, all the animals and insects, and fish, and birds, in the world, is that they consume every single particle of their diet *raw* – as it comes in nature.

And, as explained elsewhere, animals in the wild do not suffer disease. Animals in the wild, barring injury or consuming poisons, do not become ill. Unlike us humans, riddled with chronic illness and getting worse by the generation. By the day, even!

Man used to have a much-reduced diet, when you consider the natural foods of the South Sea Islanders discussed elsewhere in this book. They ate abundantly of fruits and vegetables in their raw state, and there was no large-scale foray into cordon bleu cooking, and the massive selection of confectionery available nowadays was simply not on their radar.

There was no de-hulling of wheat to produce white flour, or the removing of the husks of natural rice to end up with the nutrient-robbed white rice. The South Sea Islanders thrived on the relatively meagre selection of foods available to them. But they were happy and contented with life.

Our white bread should rightly be called the Staff of Death and not the staff of life. White bread and white rice should similarly be described as deadly, as their nutrient-packed outer husks have been removed to suit the requirements of the global food industry.

In Alfred McCann's *The Science of Eating* (1918),[18] he states:

"In May 1912, I received from the honourable secretary of the Bread and Food Reform League of England a record of the experiments conducted by Dr Frederick Gowland Hopkins, Fellow of the Royal Society, reader in chemical physiology of the University of Cambridge.

Hopkins experimented with an 80 percent whole wheat meal, which, though not containing all of the wheat, yet retained a much larger proportion of the bran and germ than white flour.

Even with such semi-impoverished material, the results of his investigations were so remarkable that they inspired a belated agitation on behalf of whole meal loaf, or, as it was called by the London Daily Mail, "household bread".

At the same time, Dr E. S. Eddie and Dr G. C. Simpson, members of the research staff at the School of Tropical Medicine, University of Liverpool, carried on investigations in which the effects of refined flour and white bread upon children and adults were carefully studied in contrast with the effects of whole meal or whole wheat bread.

The results afford further irrefutable evidence of the essential health-giving qualities of those parts of grain and cereal foods which are discarded in the milling of flour (to make white bread), the polishing of rice (to make white rice), the pearling of barley, refining of rye, and the degerminating of corn. One thing we know: the mountain of rejected food minerals is balanced, alas, how inadequately, by a lake of patent medicines.

Dr Frederick Gowland Hopkins will prove a stumbling block to all millers of "patent" flour. He says: "The superior value of whole wheat meal lies in the fact that it retains certain food substances whose presence allows our systems to make full use of the tissue-building elements of the grain. These substances are removed in the milling, leaving the fine white flour."

All my work to date confirms my belief in the superior food value of standard whole wheat bread. After definitely proving that young animals grow with very much greater rapidity on brown flour than on white, I have been able to improve the tissue-building rate of the white flour subjects by adding to their white flour an extract made from the brown flour.

Eddie and Simpson, research staff at the School of Tropical Medicine, University of Liverpool, said: "It has been proved by Braddon and other workers in the East that exclusive use of polished (white) rice as a diet leads to a form of acidosis or peripheral neuritis. This disease does not occur in those native races who use whole rice or unpolished rice (brown rice) as a diet.

"Our own experiments have been extended to similar work in relation to the stripping of the outer case from the wheat berry so as to produce a white bread instead of a brown bread and we find that parallel results are obtained when the outer layers are excluded from the diet with both wheat and rice.

"These experiments clearly demonstrate that the outer part of the grain contains the essential constituents for the nutrition of the nervous system, both in growing animals and adult humans."

Benjamin Moore, chief of the biochemical department of the Liverpool School of Tropical Medicine, as the result of his laboratory research, was forced to the following conclusions:

"Groups of pigeons have been fed on fine white bread made from white flour, known to be unbleached and unadulterated, while similar groups of pigeons have been given an ordinary quality of whole wheat bread.

"The white-bread pigeons have all speedily developed marked symptoms of malnutrition and serious nerve derangements. Besides losing weight, they sit listless and shivering, lose power in their legs, suggesting nerve paralysis, while many develop convulsions.

"The whole wheat bread fed pigeons, on the other hand, continue healthy and up to normal weight.

"In another series of experiments, pigeons which had developed grave nervous symptoms on a white bread diet recovered completely when, after a week of special nursing, they were placed on an exclusive whole wheat bread."

Harter states: "Three pigeons fed upon white bread and casein (the main protein of milk and cheese) lived 13, 25, and 29 days respectively. Two dogs fed upon soaked meat, fat, sugar, and white bread were at the point of death at the end of the 26th and 36th day respectively. Two other dogs, completely deprived of food, were comparatively active at the end of 40 and 60 days respectively. ... One dog fed on bread made from bleached flour died in 15 days. Another fed solely on white bread died in 24 days."

Only man has strayed so far from nature that we have effectively lost sight of how we *should* eat.

Children growing up today often have no conception of what should rightly be food and what should not. They can eat white bread with seeming impunity; they feel no different after eating it; therefore they believe it to be good – certainly safe. They see Harry eating a candy bar and Harry is still standing, still alive after doing so; so it further compounds the harmlessness of such non-foods.

Such foods, to them, do no harm. Or so they think.

The difficulty lies in getting over to children, indeed now even adults, that it is the long-term eating of such abominations that can result in future health problems.

It is only when they decide to eat naturally, returning to nature, that they will notice their illnesses retreat and health returning. If it is not too late, of course!

As stated elsewhere, animals in the wild, who eat natural foods, do not display illness. As Arnold de Vries states in *The Science of Eating*, "In its home among the trees, the monkey is ignorant of the meaning of processed foods. No hunter ever captured a monkey in its natural habitat suffering from appendicitis, tuberculosis, tumours, or swollen glands. ... Remove the monkey from its natural home and its natural food and the superintendent of the menagerie will bury it before its time."

He continues: "Come with me to the zoological gardens in Bronx Park and see for yourself what happens to the chimpanzee in captivity. All the primates die before their time. Tuberculosis, pneumonia, tumours, kill them."

6.

The Folly of Cooked Foods

Among the first scientists to study cooking food in its application to animal nutrition were Weill and Mouriquand of France.

In 1912, as they were conducting their celebrated experiments with pigeons to determine the effects of refined (white) flour, they added a lesser known series of experiments, also with pigeons, to determine the effects of cooking.

A number of pigeons were fed whole raw grains; the others were given the same kind of grain, entirely whole, without any kind of refining, only this grain was heated – thoroughly cooked.

The pigeons given the raw grain showed great activity and vigour. They gave every indication of being perfectly nourished. Those given the cooked grains developed beriberi and all died paralysed within 90 days.

Other pigeons were then given two-thirds cooked grain and one-third raw grain, which was sufficient to give complete freedom from what were shown to be beriberi symptoms.

Cooking our foods is such an ordinary occurrence that I can understand how extremely difficult it might be to accept the very idea that eating cooked foods can be harmful. And if we, as adults, find it hard to take on board, how much more difficult is it for our children?

The difficulty is in the immediacy of results that we come to expect.

You can smoke cigarettes for many years and still be alive and apparently well. That in itself would have made it very difficult to persuade people back in the 1930s, when smoking was considered "cool" or "sophisticated", that it could be harmful, even fatal.

So it is with food. The fact you can consume a cooked meal and, instead of dropping down dead, feel a sensation of well-being at such a lovely feast, further makes the connection between food and illness just that much more difficult to conceive.

However, just as with cigarettes and alcohol, it is the long-term results that will determine your later health; or, in more and more cases nowadays, even the health of your teenage years.

Humans have eaten cooked foods for hundreds of years. But they have also had illnesses for hundreds of years. We consider arthritis as being an ailment of old age; we consider it the "price" we have to pay for reaching an old age. But many people reach old age without arthritis. And nowadays even children are falling victim to this debilitating condition.

Heart disease and cancer are two more conditions, previously rare, but now all too common. Both of these are linked to what we put into that hole in our heads – whether it be inhaled tobacco or poor nutrition.

Furthermore, the enormous – and increasing – variety of "foods" available to us, which are really not foods at all, but confectionery or some other concoctions, are also adding to the toxic load pouring into our bodies. These are a million miles away from what we were intended to eat. But enjoy them we do, which makes the connection to ill health all the more difficult, and virtually impossible, to convey to our children.

And, as the chapter on the Pottenger Cats' study shows, each subsequent generation of animals fed on a cooked food diet develops more and more health problems. Therefore, common sense would suggest that human health will also be affected by the diets of our forefathers. By eating modern foodstuffs – highly processed and denatured – we are almost certainly building up problems for future generations.

Even the soil on which our food grows is more deficient, more poisoned now than it has ever been. Artificial fertilisers and toxic chemicals sprayed on the ground – these are simply not natural. And whilst we might not consider them to be harmful to the soil, we only believe that because we know no better. The soil will not be getting the natural nourishment it should.

If the soil is not properly nourished, then the produce that grows from that soil will be deficient in some, or many, of the nutrients that *should* be present in them. Consequently, when we eat that produce, our bodies will be deprived of vital vitamins, minerals, enzymes and other nutrients, not to mention others that still have yet to be discovered.

The lack of immediacy of symptoms lulls us all into a false sense of security when eating. We experience no immediate illness, therefore we consider that meal completely harmless.

Much as we would dearly miss our cooked meals if we were to adopt a raw diet, the fact remains that, if eating raw foods is what is required to restore an ill body to health, then we cannot argue with Nature. If our body demands such a nutritional approach, then our body demands it, whether we like it or not.

You need not necessarily have to stick rigidly to an all-raw diet. The Gerson therapy, which you will read about later, is a nearly all-raw diet that has the satisfaction of hot soups and baked potatoes, which can provide a pleasant compromise for our jaded, cooked-food palates.

Although we may have been eating cooked foods for thousands of years, it does not mean to say we have been right. Before man discovered fire, he ate as Nature intended. And that was raw.

On that raw diet primitive man would flourish, disease-free, living a long, happy, and satisfying life.

That flies in the face of those who state that primitive man lived a short life, developed bad teeth, with many health conditions, and died young. The evidence in this book will show that the very opposite is true!

You have to realise that when man was first put on Earth – by whatever means, but there had to be a first man or group of men – he would have had nothing but the land, and whatever grew from it, to eat.

If he could not subsist on whatever foliage or fruit there was, then he would hunt for animals.

Now, you don't have to be a believer in God to recognise that we have all been designed by some superior intelligence. That has to be a "given".

Do you think that such an intelligence, capable of producing the impossibly-complex and perfect body of a human, would not also design the perfect foods for that perfect body?

And that food, way back then, was raw foliage, vegetation, fruits, vegetables, nuts, and yes, even the occasional animal if the rest were not available, although our body's physiology is similar to an ape, which is not a meat eater.

Man in primitive times is still the same physiologically as man today. But we now have inferior health because of our appalling diets and our parents' and grandparents' health would have a bearing on our own. This can be seen in the story of the Pottenger Cats study, further on.

However, you can still turn your health around, the speed of which is down to you – whether you choose to go all out for it and eat completely raw and organic (not sprayed with poisons), or part-raw.

7.

Can We Extend Our Lifespan?

Applying the general animal experience with raw food to man, we may expect, therefore, to see a greater increase in the average lifespan and a considerable improvement in the state of health.

On the former point we must speculate, though with good biological foundation, as a completely raw diet has not yet been used throughout life, under scientific observation, by any member of the human race.

But an extended lifespan for those animals on a raw diet suggests that the same may be possible for man, though more than one generation might be required and other hygienic factors may also enter the picture.

What, one may ask, would the optimum length of human life be under such conditions, as nutrition became adequate and all biological requirements were successfully met?

What would be our lifespan if our parents both ate raw from the day they were born to the day they died, and if their own parents before them ate the same way, and their parents before them?

We can only speculate, but all the evidence suggests we would be in superb health, and live a far longer lifespan than we currently experience.

Man's *intended* lifespan may be considerably more than we currently consider normal. The true intended age might approximate to 100 or 150 years. We know that there have been the occasional human who has lived to 120 or beyond.

Jeanne Calment, who died in August 1997, claimed to have met the artist Vincent van Gogh (1853-1890) in Aries, where she lived. The French lady reached the grand old age of 122 years and 164 days by the time of her death. So it is eminently clear that the human body is *capable* of living to 122 years *at least*.

What would be the lifespan of someone living and eating raw – as clearly they have been designed to live and eat? One can only speculate, but the lessons we learn from animals and primitive man suggest that we are living, at present, woefully short of our potential lifespans.

Haller, the great physiologist of the 18th century, gave an even higher estimate and considered man's normal span of life to be no less than 200 years. Hufeland agreed and claimed that man's organism "is capable of living and functioning to the age of 200 years".

The scientist Elie Metchnikoff was more conservative, though his estimate of more than a century as the normal limit of human life indicated a great increase over the present-day life expectancy.

After 15 years of research on the subject, the late Alexander A. Bogomolets, founder and director of the Kief Institute of Experimental Biology in the Soviet Ukraine, issued this viewpoint: "It may sound paradoxical, but a man of 60 or 70 is still young. He has lived only half his natural life. ... Normal longevity at the present level of human development may be scientifically determined as being 125 to 150 years. There is no reason, however, to consider these figures as limits."

Thomas Parr did not marry until he was 80. He remained a farmer until he was 130, being able, until that time, to plough and thrash. He died in 1635 at the age of 152. His last days were spent in the luxurious court of Charles I, and the change in his diet is supposed to have hastened his end. His remains were dissected by Harvey, the King's physician and noted discoverer of the circulation of the blood, and showed no signs of decay in any organs. His diet on the farm he ploughed was simple and came from the land.

Parr was treated as a spectacle in London, but the change in food and environment apparently led to his death. The king arranged for him to be buried in Westminster Abbey on 15 November 1635. The inscription on his gravestone reads:[19]

THO: PARR OF YE COUNTY OF SALLOP.
BORNE IN AD: 1483.
HE LIVED IN YE REIGNES OF TEN PRINCES VIZ:
K.ED.4. K.ED.5. K.RICH.3. K.HEN.7. K.HEN.8.
K.EDW.6. Q.MA. Q.ELIZ., K.JA. & K. CHARLES.
AGED 152 YEARES. & WAS BURYED HERE
NOVEMB. 15. 1635.

One does wonder, if our children today were brought up from the outset on raw foods from an early age, to what age might they live? Perhaps the idea of Methuselah reaching 900 years in the bible might not be such a ridiculous consideration after all. If our bodies can live to 123, and in Parr's case, 152, who knows what long life we may have if we were to apply nature's dietary rules.

On the relationship of raw food to the length of human life, we may thus arrive at an optimistic biological probability. On the relationship of raw food to the development of specific diseases, and the treatment of specific diseases, we can also be optimistic, though in this case we need not speculate at all, but can cite many human experiences which afford corroboration.

Fortunately, there has been very extensive human use of certain raw foods in certain areas, and there has been much clinical work done already with exclusive raw-food diets.

These show, in actual practice, exactly to what extent the animal experiences with raw food can be applied to humans, pertaining to physical development and the prevalence of many common diseases.

8.

The Health of Wild Animals

Animals, in wild nature, do not suffer the illnesses that man is prey to. They forage for their own, specific, foods. And they do not suffer from chronic health conditions like man. They eventually die from starvation, lack of water, injury – whether from another animal or a fall – but they simply do not have the array of health disorders that man with his cooked-to-death food has.

The biologist, Sir J. Arthur Thompson, has often referred to the healthfulness of nature as being manifested by the absence of senility and the rarity of more than mild senescence. He states that man has "a monopoly on senility" and in wild nature "there may be indications of senescence or normal ageing, but there is no senility".

It is difficult to tell the age of some mature animals without examining the teeth for wear. After maturity is reached, the ageing process is very slow, and all animals look very much alike. A decrepit animal is so rare that few naturalists, hunters, or trappers ever see one. As Thompson so well points out: "Nature has much more to teach man than he has yet learned, and it would be well, indeed, if man could come closer to wild nature's standard of positive health and prolonged youthfulness."

In the animal world, the primates are man's closest relative from the standpoint of comparative anatomy and physiology. Their excellent health and longevity whilst living on raw foods in their natural habitat are of special importance to us. According to the naturalist, Barnes, the gorillas live in nature a "life free from molestation, famine, or disease, also judging by the worn teeth of one animal I secured, they live, in my opinion, to [a] much greater age than man."

On the authority of the primitive Dyaks of Borneo, who are in the best position to know, the orangutan lives in the wild fully 40 to 50 years *longer* than man, and it is not seen to suffer from any disease in its life.

Chimpanzees, gibbons, and baboons have a shorter lifespan, though they live far longer in the wild than they do in captivity, and they are quite free from the symptoms of senility. Indeed, explorers and hunters in Africa very rarely report seeing a senile primate. The gorilla has been seen to lose a part of pigmentation of hair in advanced years – resulting in the "silverback" – though this is an indication of normal senescence rather than the pathology of senility.

The health and vigour in wild nature is, judging from all evidence, due in the main to the consumption of completely natural, raw foods. The exclusive raw-food diet is the norm of all wildlife. When man's interference does not place into existence compensatory factors, it is associated with a relatively high level of physical excellence.

When an animal is placed in captivity or domestication, with the continued use of raw foods, it continues to maintain this physical excellence in spite of the limited compensatory factors that may be present. If the animal is given heat-processed, or cooked, foods, it fails to maintain its normal forms of immunity, and often fails to survive, even though all the other factors – exercise, rest, sunshine, pure air, freedom to move, etc – are favourable.

9.

Raw Foods in Humans

Can the results of animal experience be successfully applied to humans? The basic importance of food to the existence and health of any living organisms, whether it be man, or insect, or elephant, must be recognised as obvious. The experiments and studies in this book must surely heap all the more importance on such a relationship.

If it is possible to use the information gleaned from animal studies and transfer it to humans, then food will be seen to be the most important single factor in determining the state of human health.

The research – both human and animal – throughout this book should offer hope to the "incurably" sick, as every indicator is that by applying the same approach – a raw diet as opposed to a cooked one – then the sick can regain health. This book should also offer hope to the present system of medicine that is currently – and always has been – groping in the dark when it comes to curing human disease and physical degeneration.

But will our system of medicine even *look* at such studies, far less take guidance from them? They have not, thus far.

Biologists believe that the greater part of animal experience in the use of foods can be applied to humans. They point out that man is governed by the same basic biological and physiological laws that exist throughout the animal kingdom.

Whether or not man is placed on a different mental or spiritual level than other forms of animal life, no scientist would attempt to place him on a different physical level.

When experimental animals are given a diet similar to that of various human racial groups, their physical condition and rate of disease often correspond almost exactly with that of humans using the same foods.

This was best demonstrated by Sir Robert McCarrison in India. He placed groups of white rats on diets which corresponded to those of racial groups in India and other parts of the world. He found that rats given the diets of the relatively healthy people of India – Hunzas, Sikhs, and Pathans – attained the same good health these peoples attained.

Those rats fed the diets of the less healthy Indian races failed to maintain their physical vigour and suffered from disease at the same rate that the respective people did. For instance, the rats fed a cooked and refined diet similar to that used in the Indian city of Madras developed ulcers in 10 percent of all cases, which corresponds exactly with the percentage of ulcers among the inhabitants of the province.

For those given the cooked foods of the Travancorian area, the rate of ulcers was 25 percent, just as it is among the Travancorian people. Fifty percent of the rats on the Sind diet developed stones in the bladder, and half of the people in the Sind province suffer from the same ailment.

Such striking similarity in the reaction of man and other animals to various foods applies in the main to the forms of processing the food undergoes, not to the specific kind of food itself. All animals, including man, do not react exactly the same way to a strictly carnivorous, insectivorous, omnivorous, herbivorous, or frugivorous diet.

Each animal has certain dietary limitations, determined by physiology and anatomy, which must be met. Members of the cat family, for instance, would not get along on a diet of grass with the same efficiency as hoofed mammals; nor could the latter animals secure adequate nutrition by using animal flesh exclusively.

However, with each animal group, including the higher primate, adhering to its normal dietary customs, but having the same percentage of foods cooked and refined, there is remarkable resemblance in the kind of disease developed, its intensity, and the general physical development as a whole.

This does not mean that every animal experiment can be applied, in all particulars, to man; but a general application is almost always possible.

Man can achieve a relatively high immunity to some diseases, if much of the diet remains raw. And the ill-effects of a cooked diet appear to take longer with man than they do with animals. Man, having lived mostly upon cooked foods for hundreds of years, does not always experience the violent reactions that a wild animal or experimental animal that is given cooked foods for the first time, will do.

10.

Sir Robert McCarrison

Whilst Director of Nutrition Research under the Research Fund Association in India, the celebrated British scientist, Sir Robert McCarrison, carried out experiments in nutrition after having visited a remote tribe called the Hunzas, who displayed superb health and longevity. Their freedom from disease was remarkable and the men worked in the fields well into their 90s.

McCarrison was so convinced that their health was down to their mostly raw, natural food diet and the pure water from the glaciers, that he decided to conduct experiments on white rats with raw and cooked foods.

McCarrison set up the first large-scale experiments with white rats which revealed the effects of cooking. One thousand pedigree albino rats were placed on a diet of raw cabbage, raw carrots, raw milk, raw meat, unleavened bread, and sprouted legumes.[20]

Two thousand rats were then placed on a diet of white bread, margarine, tinned meat, tinned jam, boiled tea, boiled potatoes, boiled cabbage, and a small amount of milk.

All animals were given the same general care. The laboratory was kept perfectly clean; the tiled floor and walls were frequently washed. The cages were large and spacious, so each rat could run about and exercise as it pleased.

The rats given primarily raw foods were remarkably healthy in all respects. From all appearances they suffered from no diseases whatsoever, and all mothers reared their young. At the end of two and a quarter years, corresponding to 55 years in man, all rats were autopsied. The only trace of disease found was an occasional cyst in the liver, which was assumed due to the straw bedding which the rats often nibbled.

The 2,000 rats eating mostly cooked foods soon began developing a wide assortment of diseases – practically every ailment that one might find listed in any medical textbook!

Foremost among these, as revealed in the post-mortem examinations, were: tuberculosis, arthritis, Bright's disease, gastric ulcers, duodenal ulcers, glandular enlargements, inflammation of the eyes, anaemia, loss of hair, infected teeth, infected tonsils, middle-ear disease, corneal ulceration, and skin diseases of various types.

In addition, the rats seemed to be affected mentally. In contrast to the raw-food rats, which were gentle and affectionate, these animals became ill-tempered and vicious. They would bite the attendant, kill each other, and generally display a state of continuous nervous irritability.

Following the rat experiments, McCarrison used 20 monkeys in a new series of tests. All animals except one were in perfect condition when the experiment began – the exception being the result of a slight injury sustained by one monkey during capture.

Nine of the monkeys were placed on a diet consisting chiefly of raw foods, including wheaten bread, milk, ground nuts, fresh onions, fresh butter, plantains, and water.

Six were given wheaten bread, cooked rice, cooked ground nuts, boiled milk, fresh butter, and water.

The other five were given a similar assortment of cooked foods, fresh onions and water, plus a little fresh butter.

All animals were provided with the same amount of exercise, sunshine, fresh air, etc. The only difference in their mode of life was their diet, involving the condition (cooked or raw) in which the food was given.

Regarding the monkeys fed primarily raw foods, McCarrison stated:

"They remained in good health, with the exception of an attack of jaundice in some of them; this was thought to be due to the sudden lack of exercise, as well as to the too generous provision of monkey-nuts, which in the earlier stages of the experiment were not limited to 10 grams.

The jaundice was corrected by reducing the diet to milk and bananas for a few days, and adding magnesium sulphate to the drinking water. After recovery, which occurred in all cases, the diet, as above-detailed, was used without recurrence of jaundice or any untoward symptoms whatsoever."

The monkeys given cooked foods developed troubles from the very start. Diseases were common and every animal died within 43 to 100 days. Average length of life of those given the cooked foods plus onions was 60 days. Those allowed a little butter each day lived an average of 69 days.

The post-mortems of these monkeys indicated the presence of dozens of physical abnormalities and ailments.

These included: dilation of the stomach, gastric catarrh, stomach ulcers, duodenal catarrh, degeneration of the mucous membrane, congestive changes in the jejunum and ileum, ballooning of the small bowel, atrophy and thinning of the walls of the small intestine, colitis, ballooning of the colon, atrophy of the omentum, and cancer of the pylorus.

OTHER ANIMAL EXPERIMENTS WITH RAW FOOD

Experiments with guinea pigs, to determine the effects of cooked foods, were conducted by Dr O. Steiner, an investigator for the Swiss Board of Health, in Berne, Switzerland. Dr Steiner placed a large group of these animals on a diet of their normal foods (hay, oats, carrots, and water), which would normally be taken raw, but in this case were cooked in a high-pressure steamer. A large number of diseases appeared shortly thereafter.

The teeth became softened to such an extent that they could be cut away with scissors. Gangrenous gingivitis developed, and the jaws softened and warped until the rows of teeth overlapped and would not close in the normal manner.

The salivary glands became diseased and the animals developed both goitre and anaemia. In certain cases, two teaspoons of pasteurised milk each day were added to the diet, and this was followed by the development of another disease, arthritis. Most of the guinea pigs died of scurvy, with a smaller number succumbing to cancer of the lung.

Dried skimmed milk had been heralded as a "super food" in some quarters, but experimental animals live very poorly on this food after it has been heat-processed during manufacture or at any other time. Dr Joseph E. Muller, of Indiana University, found that white rats given unheated dried milk had only 5.4 percent dental defects, whilst the caries incidence rose to 9.3 percent when heated dried milk was given.

McClure and Folk likewise found that dried milk produced dental caries in rats, with the amount of damage being parallel with the degree of heating the milk had undergone.

Kraft and Morgan, of the University of California, reported that the dried milk lost half of its growth efficiency for rats if it had been cooked for 15 minutes, and all of its growth value if cooked for 25 minutes.

From Germany comes a report from Fink and Schlie, who tested 21 samples of dried skimmed milk as contrasted to fresh skimmed milk. Of 200 rats given the dried milk, 95 percent died within 40 to 100 days, and 85 percent of these had liver necrosis.

All rats given the same diet, but with fresh skimmed milk instead of dried milk, survived the experiment with complete freedom from liver necrosis.[21]

Cats and dogs fed commercial pet foods which have all been heat-processed show various symptoms of disease in experimental tests. M. L. Morris fed a group of cats on fresh meat and all thrived well, but those animals given samples of many different commercial cat foods did poorly in comparison, and a number of the cats showed emaciation, skin lesions, and neurological signs.

Dr Clive McCay has pointed out that, "The meat meals commonly used in dog feeds are often so over-heated in processing that they are entirely devoid of vitamin B1."

In a digestion trial of meat meals made by students, the dog refused to eat and became badly constipated. Koehn observed that dogs may appear healthy and thrive for long periods on cooked rations containing cottonseed meal, "but eventually they will die very suddenly".

Dogs fed upon raw foods are resistant to experimental amoebic infection, but those animals given a diet of canned meat have very low resistance.

E. C. Foust found that he could produce amoebic infection at will in poorly nourished animals and then establish a cure by feeding them raw liver. This food arrested the amoebic lesion and at the same time lessened the danger of secondary bacterial infection.

Magendie made extensive feeding trials with dogs to determine the effects of raw bones. Animals given boiled bones died within a couple of months, and those fed the heat-processed bone extract, gelatin, for a few days, preferred to die rather than eat more. Fresh raw bones, on the other hand, kept the dogs alive for long periods and appeared to afford adequate nourishment.

The canine experience with milk has been much the same. An English physician reported feeding puppies on pasteurised milk, and the animals died. Other puppies were given raw milk and thrived well. The American physician, Dr Charles Sanford, reported that, "Dogs fed on pasteurised milk only are liable to have the mange and other disorders, while others of the same litter thrive on raw, sweet and sour milk".

11.

Raw Milk vs Pasteurised Milk

Today's scientists have it badly wrong with many aspects of human nutrition, not least of which is milk.

They assume that heating the milk – pasteurising it – will kill bacteria and any organisms that may threaten human health. They assume, therefore, that pasteurised milk will be better for our health.

The truth is quite different, and it puts to shame the fact that such people should be in any way in charge of human nutrition.

We are expected to blindly respect everything that is "scientific". But history, and even the present time, is testament to the gross errors of judgement scientists can make in the manner in which we consume our food.

Much of the studies of raw food consumption involve studying raw versus pasteurised milk. As soon as pasteurisation came into use, striking changes were observed in public health statistics, particularly with regard to infants.

In the first part of the 20th century, in the three largest hospitals in Toronto, Canada, there was a sharp increase in the death rate after pasteurised milk came into use.

In Berlin, Germany, pasteurisation was adopted in 1901, and was followed by a virtual epidemic of scurvy throughout the city, though previously this disease was uncommon.

An investigation was made as to the cause of the disease; pasteurisation was judged responsible, and, as the process was later discontinued, the scurvy disappeared just as rapidly as it had appeared.

In 1917, the American scientist, Dr A. E. Hess, of Columbia University, published the results of his extensive research on the cause and remedy of scurvy.[22]

He indicated that scurvy could be produced or cured at will in infants simply by altering their diet with regard to the use of raw and pasteurised milk.

Infants given only pasteurised milk tended to display evidence of scurvy within six months.

Those on raw milk were free from the disease; and when the food was added to the diet of those already afflicted, recovery was the general rule.

Subsequent investigations by Ragnar Berg and other scientists have confirmed the experience of Hess.

Scurvy is now universally recognised to be a deficiency disease which can be prevented by the use of raw milk or other food of adequate potency in the vitamin C content, such as limes, or other citrus fruits.

In the 1930s, Dr Evelyn Sprawson, of the London Hospital, studied the rate of dental decay among children in orphanages and found that the percentage of decay varied in direct proportion to the amounts of raw or pasteurised milk in their diet.[23]

Children in institutions that used only raw milk had excellent teeth as contrasted to others.

Among 750 boys in one institution, the addition of a daily ration of raw milk to the diet caused a marked reduction in the number of caries, the effects being noticeable within two to three years after the beginning of milk feeding.

Data was collected regarding 40 children – aged 2 to 7 – who received raw milk regularly from the age of four and a half months and exhibited complete absence of caries.

Another group of 58 was examined who received raw milk regularly from the age of six years, and they showed no caries in any tooth erupted after this period.

A third group, which started taking raw milk at the age of ten years, showed good results.

It was noted that all teeth that had erupted, but were not yet fully formed, came under the beneficial influence of raw milk.

Of further interest is the fact that the children given raw milk attained improved general health over the others. Fewer of them required tonsil and adenoid operations, as compared with other children, which suggests an improvement in the quality of lymphoid tissue throughout the body.

Bone development among infants and children has long been known to be dependent upon the use of raw or pasteurised milk.

The incidence of rickets rose 100 percent in the city of Baltimore,

Maryland, when pasteurised milk was introduced as standard food for infants in the city.

Raw milk in itself affords freedom from rickets, though pasteurised milk must be balanced with certain other foods or fish liver oil supplements if protection is to be provided.

Special pasteurised milk, to which a certain amount of vitamin D has been added through the process of irradiation, may prevent rickets, but it has been proven to be very detrimental to animals in other ways, and Dr Steiner has reported that it may also prove harmful to non-rachitic children.[24]

The prevalence of certain infectious diseases also appears to depend to some extent upon the type of milk used in the diet. Investigators have pointed out that gripe and diphtheria occur more frequently among infants given pasteurised milk, especially when it forms the predominant part of the diet.

Digestion, too, is more difficult when pasteurised milk is used. Cohen and Ruelle, of the Department of Paediatrics, in the University of Brussels, employed raw milk with good results in the treatment of specific digestive disturbances.

In the case of diarrhoea and vomiting, they gave small amounts of raw milk every 1 to 2 hours to promote recovery. They believe that certain ferments in milk which aid digestion are destroyed by heating.[25]

Milk tests among children in schools in Scotland have been made which indicated that both weight and height increases among children were dependent upon the form of milk that was used.

Fisher and Bartlett have analysed the figures resulting from these tests. They have expressed the relative value of pasteurised milk as a percentage of that of raw milk, as demonstrated by increases in weight and height when the latter is used.

Listing the increase on raw milk as 100 percent, they show that on pasteurised milk the weight increase for boys was only 66 percent, in girls 91 percent. For height, the increase in boys was 50 percent and 70 percent in girls, the increase thus being significantly greater for both sexes, in terms of weight and height, when raw milk was used.[26]

Another study, by Perkin and Strachan of St. George's University of London,[27] showed a link between consumption of raw, unpasteurised milk and a lowered prevalence of allergies. The study also showed that raw milk consumption was associated with significantly less current eczema symptoms.

Dr Frances Pottenger, Jr, whilst best known for his animal studies with raw and pasteurised milk (which are described elsewhere in this book), has also tested these foods on a clinical basis.

He reports that infants fed on raw milk tend to be healthy, whereas those given standard formulae consisting of powdered milk, pasteurised milk, boiled milk, canned milk, etc, frequently suffer from gastric distress, asthma, respiratory infections, bronchitis, and colds.

X-rays of raw milk-fed infants revealed densely mineralised bones of adequate thickness, together with wide chests and broad dental arches. X-rays of the infants given heat-processed milk showed thin and fragile bones, abnormal mineral deposits, narrow chests, and underdeveloped dental arches.[28]

Dr Kirkpatrick ascribes the development of enlarged hearts, with valvular involvement, in many cases to the use of pasteurised milk.

Some of the children are said to rapidly recover if raw milk is substituted for the pasteurised milk.

"Without raw milk, recovery does not occur," declares Dr Kirkpatrick, "and those who reach the age of 10 or 15 will, upon examination, show chronic heart diseases which are usually diagnosed as rheumatic fever; so the patient usually goes through life a semi-invalid. I personally know of many children, who were suffering from heart complications, who have made complete recovery in a few months by drinking raw milk along with other wholesome foods, and with no direct treatment to the heart."[29]

In New York, studies of the relative weight gains made by infants fed pasteurised and raw milk were made by M. Ludd, H. W. Ewarts, and L. W. Franks.

The infants were divided into four groups.

The first was given only pasteurised milk; the second was given pasteurised milk plus orange juice; the third was given pasteurised milk plus orange juice and cod liver oil; and the fourth was given only raw milk.

An analysis of the percentage in weight gains made by the four groups showed that the first gained 1.7 percent in weight; the second group gained 1.7 percent; the third group gained 9.5 percent; whilst the fourth group, fed entirely upon raw milk, gained 14 percent in weight.

Contrary to popular belief, raw milk affords greater resistance to both undulant fever and typhoid fever than does pasteurised milk.

Undulant fever (brucellosis) appeared to be more common in large cities, where pasteurisation was a requirement, than in rural areas, where some raw milk was used.

Madsen of Denmark has indeed stated that, "no case [of undulant fever] has ever been observed in the hospitals and asylums for children in Copenhagen or elsewhere where raw milk is used in large quantities".

RAW MILK STUDIES IN ANIMALS

In America, Dr Rosalind Wulzen and Alice Bahrs, of the Department of Zoology in Oregon State College, used guinea pigs in their experimental work. Efforts were made to determine the effects of pasteurised milk. The animals were divided into four groups, which were given raw milk, pasteurised milk, raw skimmed milk, and pasteurised skimmed milk, respectively.

"Animals fed raw whole milk grew excellently and an autopsy showed no abnormality of any kind," Dr. Wulzen reported. Animals fed pasteurised milk did not grow as well, and developed stiffness of the muscles. Within a period of a month to a year they died, after showing signs of "great emaciation and weakness". The autopsy revealed that the muscles were extremely atrophied and streaked with white lines of calcification. Lumps of tricalcium phosphate were found deposited under the skin, in the joints, the heart, and other organs.

In addition to guinea pigs, white rats were used in the tests at Oregon State College, these being reported by Bahrs and Hughes. The animals given pasteurised milk gained weight less rapidly than those given raw milk, and on autopsy the hearts were found to have a flabby appearance. The adrenal glands were of a pale colour and there were small areas of apparent atrophy. The livers and skeletal muscles also exhibited a very pale colour, as compared to those of the animals given raw milk.

At Ohio State University, Dr Ernest Scott and Prof Lowell Erf also fed different groups of rats on raw and pasteurised milk. The animals on raw milk showed a good, sleek coat; they were adequate in growth and weight; their eyes were clear; their dispositions were excellent, and they enjoyed being petted.

Those on pasteurised milk had a roughened coat; their growth was slow; their eyes lacked lustre; and they were very irritable, often showing a tendency to bite when being handled. The rats on pasteurised milk also showed a loss of vitality and weight, and many developed anaemia.

Using rats in a similar set of experiments, Scott and Erf noted the following results when pasteurised milk was used as a partial ration for the animals: "(a) Incomplete mineralisation of the offspring. (b) The inability of the animal to remineralise its own skeleton adequately after pregnancy and likely to produce a rachitic condition in the offspring. (c) Failure in the development of the teeth. (d) Muscular and ligamentous atony as well as changes in the histological factor of the various organs. (e) Tendency toward development in allergies. (f) Tendency toward sterility in subsequent generations.[30]

Two English scientists, Mattick and Golding, employed white rats in a series of experiments, also with milk. They fed different groups of the animals fresh raw milk, pasteurised milk, and sterilised milk. Those receiving raw milk attained normal weight and growth in each of the four generations the experiments were conducted. Rats receiving pasteurised milk grew less rapidly, and reproduction was impaired. The animals given sterilised milk grew less rapidly than either of the other two groups; reproduction was also less efficient, and none of the animals in the third generation lived longer than a day.

Another investigator, S. S. Schmidt-Nielson, fed white rats pasteurised milk and reported that the food produced diminished vitality and early death in the offspring of mature animals. Daniels and Loughlin reported the failure of normal growth in all rats given heated milk, whether evaporated, condensed, or pasteurised.

They also observed that this milk increased the tendency of the animals to develop polyneuritis.

Given adequate amounts of raw milk, none of the animals developed this disease; whereas three on pasteurised milk were severely afflicted.

Kitchin and McFarland noted that raw milk provided good growth curves in rats; whereas growth among animals given pasteurised milk was poor.

Russell observed that the addition of raw beef to a wheat-milk diet in rats improved reproduction and increased the general vigour of the young.

Abeline reported that rats fed whole wheat bread baked at high temperatures were stunted in growth and not so resistant to disease as were rats given bread baked at low temperatures.

In Finland, Dr Reinius reported feeding rats a diet composed exclusively of food heated in an oven at 140 degrees C for 30 or 40 minutes. This caused total cessation of growth of the animals, which was attributed to the destruction of certain amino acids by heat.

McCandlish and Black, of the West of Scotland College of Agriculture, tested raw and pasteurised milk on the growth and health of calves. Fourteen calves of different breeds and sexes were divided into two groups of six and eight, respectively, one receiving raw milk from the age of five days and the other receiving pasteurised milk from the same age.

At the end of 60 days, all calves on raw milk were alive and in good health. Of those on pasteurised milk, two had died and one had to be removed on account of "unthriftiness". For the first 60 days there was no significant difference in the rate of growth, but after that period the calves on raw milk grew more rapidly. The calves on pasteurised milk consumed more food per pound of weight gained, using 6 percent more milk, 16 percent more grain, and 43 percent more hay.

W. Catel, using goats, also found better results from the use of raw milk. Animals so fed attained much better growth than those using pasteurised milk, though some fared badly when given milk from the bottle, but thrived well on the mother's milk obtained naturally. Catel found that, "The utilisation of fat, carbohydrate, protein, calcium, and phosphorous was less complete in the animals fed on heated milk; these animals retained a very high proportion of choline in their food."

The famous epidemic of typhoid fever in Montreal during 1927, in which there were 5,353 cases and 400 deaths, was restricted entirely to families who purchased milk from the Montreal Dairy and its associated National Dairy Company, both of which distributed only pasteurised milk.

Astonishingly, raw milk has been banned in Scotland for at least 20 years, but is allowed just across the border, in England.

12.

Psoriasis

One of the many conditions that medicine is unable to cure, or even find the cause of, is psoriasis.

"It is a chronic immune-mediated disease that appears on the skin. It occurs when the immune system apparently sends out faulty signals that speed up the growth cycle of skin cells," says the medical literature.

But can it be cured by a raw diet?

Dr George Clements was an American medical doctor who grew more and more discouraged at his inability to help his patients with the methods he had at his disposal, and eventually studied Orthopathy and Nature Cure, gaining a real insight for the first time into disease and its causes.

In their book on *Orthopathy*,[31] Drs Shelton and Clements reported that natural food, in less than three months, cured a serious case of psoriasis of 28 years standing – and this after years of all sorts and kinds of medical treatment had been tried and failed.

They stated:

"When man wakes up to the fact that he breathes, drinks, and eats for the sole purpose of supplying building material to repair his constantly wearing and wasting frame, and then breathes, drinks, and eats for that purpose alone – when that day comes the world will be inhabited by a superior race, and doctors will disappear, for there will be no more "disease" for them to "cure". All skin disorders, from pimples to pox, are primarily the result of men eating wrong food. This fact was quite convincingly proved recently in a serious case of psoriasis of many years standing. The patient is a man of 33, and this is his story:

My name is Louis Denman. For 28 years I suffered with a skin affliction known as psoriasis. My entire body, from the top of my head to the soles of my feet, was covered with large, red blotches, which were covered with scale-like formation. I consulted many doctors, and in this way I spent much money, but my condition grew steadily worse. At one time, under a certain doctor's orders, I took so much arsenic that I nearly went blind, and was forced to stop taking it.

In November 1926, I heard of Dr G. R. Clements, and was told that he was very successful in securing marvelous results in all sorts of ailments, and especially in chronic ailments of long-standing. I also learned that he was an orthopath, that he gave no drugs, but employed only the simple agencies of Nature in his work. I was anxious to see what he could do for me. So I lost no time in going to him.

The first time I called at his office, he was out, but the next day I was more successful. Think of my surprise when I say that Dr Clements did not proceed to make the long and tiresome examination, which is the customary practice with medical men, and after which examination they apparently know less than they did before.

Dr Clements simply looked at the eruption on my arms and body, then asked me how long I had been in that condition, what I had done for it, and what my habits were as to eating, drinking, and so on.

I confessed to him that I had been a heavy eater of meats and pastries – but whoever had any idea that such have anything to do with an eruption on the skin? Do not physicians advise patients to eat plenty of good, nourishing food? And are meats and pastries not such food?

I also confessed that I smoked cigarettes – but most physicians also smoke, and would they if it were harmful? Surely smoking had nothing to do with my physical condition. And then I told him that I drank a little occasionally – but what of that? Had not whisky and alcohol been staple remedies with the medical profession for these many ages? What they use to 'cure' the sick should be useful in keeping the well from getting sick. If not, why not? If not, how can it help the ill back to health?

Does the medicine man of today not possess the same miraculous powers as the medicine man of antiquity; that he, like they, is able to set at naught the operation of Nature's Laws by the mere waving of his magic wand? Well, maybe he can do it, but he cannot make me believe it any more.

What did Dr Clements prescribe? Well, I had anticipated something wonderful, something extraordinary; so when he told me what to do, it was such a shock that I know just how Naaman must have felt, when Elisha sent a messenger unto him, saying: 'Go and wash in Jordan and be clean'. He merely advised me to eat only uncooked foods, drink only water, quit smoking and drinking, and observe all the habits of health, such as exercise, cleanliness, sunshine, etc. He told me that by these methods we build health, and that as we build health we 'cure' disease.

How simple. Why had I never thought of that before? We 'cure disease' by building health, and we destroy health by building 'disease', by bad habits. How can the average person discover anything so simple, and so profoundly true, when his mind is befogged by the absurd education of the age, which teaches that 'disease' results from germs, chilly winds, dampness, pollen from various wild flowers, and so on?

We build disease by bad habits, and we build health by good habits, and as we build health we 'cure' disease, or as we build disease we destroy health. That rule, or that law, whichever you care to call it, will never be 'discovered' and recognized by any school of healing, for schools of healing are searching for 'cures' for disease, and not for health-building-rules.

I can see now as I never could before, that if health-building-rules were as well and widely known as musical and mathematical rules, diseases would soon disappear, and doctors along with them, since there would be nothing for doctors to do.

Yes, Dr Clements ordered me to eat no more cooked foods – to my great surprise. Who ever heard of cooked foods being detrimental to the body? But I see it all now. There are no exceptions to Nature's Laws. Of all animals, man alone subsists on cooked foods. And observe his degenerated condition physically, mentally, morally.

Dr Clements advised me to select my food from substances that grow above the ground. Another good rule. Things that grow under ground, such as roots and tubers, have no more vitality than pot plants placed and left in cellars and dark corners of dark houses. And yet think of the vast quantities of potatoes, turnips, beets, carrots, and parsnips that people eat. A bushel of apples contains five times as much nourishment for the body as a bushel of potatoes, and a man eats a bushel of potatoes to every apple he eats.

Leafy vegetables, melons, berries, grapes, and fruits, says Dr Clements, are what men should eat if they are interested in having good health. And I was so convinced with the soundness and saneness of his argument, that I left his office feeling like a fool because I had lived all these years and had not found the simple truths which he expounded to me so clearly in less than an hour's time.

The 45 minutes that I spent in his office are really worth more to me than all the schooling and training of all the years gone by. For if a man does not know how to live to have health, what does he know that is worth a cent? For what doth it profit a man if he gain the whole world and lose his health and life? Riches can buy many things, but health and life they cannot buy.

I rigidly observed Dr Clements' advice for three long weeks – eating things I had never eaten before in that condition. Uncooked cabbage, uncooked tomatoes, and nothing on them – just the plain cabbage and tomatoes as they came from the garden. Then I ate nuts, and oranges and bananas and apples – and drank only water. For three weeks I did this – and no appreciable change could I notice. I began to grow discouraged. I reported to Dr Clements and told him that I believed he was wrong. But he urged me to stick to it a while longer. I did so at his earnest request. He appeared to have so much faith in the things he told me; and if his past experience had shown him that he was right, how could I have less faith in his advice than he had himself.

One week more passed by. Four long weeks on this diet. It seemed like a year. But the fourth week was not so bad, nor did it seem so long as the first. I was beginning to like the new diet. It did not seem to leave such a tired, heavy feeling in my stomach and bowels. A bowl of finely chopped cabbage, lettuce, and celery made me a good meal, and it seemed so light on my stomach that I did not know I had a stomach. So different from the old feeling after a heavy meal of the old style.

One more week went by, as I said – but what began to happen in that week? Could it be possible? Yes, it was true – the irritation was growing fainter, the large, ugly red blotches, which had covered my flesh from childhood, were growing paler and smaller, and the scale-like formation was gradually disappearing. The new skin was smooth and considerably clearer, and the itching burning sensation, which used to grow so marked when I perspired, was growing less and less.

When it really dawned upon me that my condition was improving, I bubbled over with joy. I called on Dr Clements and told him what was happening. I thought he would be surprised – but he wasn't.

He said that the rising of the summer sun did not surprise him, as the event is governed by a law just as fixed and certain; he said that he knew my condition would improve just as sure as the ebb and flow of the tide, provided I would follow his advice long enough. What a doctor, and what faith he has in his methods. I wish I could tell the whole world about it.

It has now been several months since my entire body has become free of that terrible affliction, which I had begun to believe I would carry to my grave, and in a very few years, had I continued to be an unthinking dupe for the medical profession. Never again will a medical man have the pleasure of extracting a dollar from my purse. I have been thru the fire and learned my lesson well. I only regret that I cannot tell what I know to millions of suffering souls.

Just one more word before I close. Never mix your food. Eat one kind of food at a meal. I mean, follow the mono-diet system, like animals do. They only eat one food at a time. When you eat vegetables, eat only vegetables; when you eat berries, eat only berries; when you eat oranges, eat only oranges; and when you eat nuts, let nuts make up the entire meal."

It should be noted that, had Louis Denman, in the above story, given up after 3 weeks of a raw diet, he would probably never have witnessed a cure to his life-long condition. In later years, if someone were to have suggested to him to try a nature cure diet, or a raw diet, he would probably have answered, "No point. I tried it before, and it failed!"

There is a great lesson to be learned from this. Recovery takes time, and no two people are alike. Louis Denman, at three weeks on the diet, was just effectively "round the corner" from the cure, and, had he given up, he would never have been free from his condition. But he persevered, and, as Dr Clements stated, he knew that his condition would improve just as sure as the ebb and flow of the tide would occur.

The diet needs three things: the raw food, perseverance, and time.

The above report of Louis Denman's recovery from "incurable" psoriasis is a report of a man's experience with a raw, natural, diet.

How else could someone, given that advice by Dr Clements, then report his recovery other than simply to report it as it happened? Yet, those with vested interests in it not being true will dismiss it, will discredit it, because they will say it is "anecdotal" and not "scientific".

How can someone who adopts a raw or any other diet in their house, and recovers, do it in such a way that it will be "scientific"? It simply is not practical to follow such instructions in an institution or hospital setting when one simply visits a doctor and is advised to adhere to a raw diet. It is simply daft to expect that. But vested interest parties will forever hang on to that "anecdotal" excuse to dismiss such stories, despite medical science having made virtually no progress at all in the past 100 years in their search for cures – for nearly any disease! You will read more on that later.

It is similar to Dr Max Gerson, who cured people with skin TB. He was taken to court by fellow physicians who specialised in skin complaints. They were furious that Gerson had success where they didn't. They wanted him charged with practising outside the boundaries of his speciality. The judgement was in Gerson's favour – the judge asked the complainers if they could cure skin TB. When they admitted they couldn't, the judge merely found in favour of Gerson.

But why would skin specialists even bother to charge Gerson when he was successful? Surely they would be happy that patients were being cured by Gerson when they had no such cure!

If only it were that simple. Personalities, pride, anger, embarrassment, shame – these all play a part in criticising recoveries by non-drug methods.

This jealousy transfers to every area of medicine. If patients can cure their own disease, expect the fury of criticisms using the terminologies of "anecdotal" or "not scientific". It is nothing but suppressed anger that they, in their own work, might not be able to achieve that success with their toxic drugs. They would have to admit that they would be barking up the wrong tree. Indeed, they *know* that they would have been barking up the wrong tree all their professional lives if the anecdotal story they have been directed to was true. No wonder they resist with all their might!

13.

We Can Heal Ourselves

Whatever illness we may suffer from, our bodies have the capacity to heal the condition.

The better the nutritional status of the body, the quicker the body will recover. The poorer the nutritional status, the slower any recovery will occur.

If the nutritional status of the body is extremely low, then the illness can gain the ascendancy and overcome the body. If we can restore the nutritional status of the body sufficiently, then good health will gain the ascendancy and defeat the disease.

We have the power within all of us to heal ourselves. It is always only our own bodies that carry out the healing of our bodies. The body strives at all times towards health. The body's normal state is one of good health. Illness is an abnormal state.

As I have stated elsewhere, we may have a cut on our finger, the nurse may well put iodine on it, and cover it with a sticking plaster. But when it heals, it will not have been healed by the iodine, nor will it have been healed by the nurse, or the sticking plaster: the body's *own*, internal, innate healing power will have achieved the repair.

It doesn't matter if it is cancer, or a broken bone, the body can repair the condition. However, the condition of the body has to be right in order to achieve healing. And the condition of the body depends on what you put into it in the way of food and drink, etc.

Animals in the wild, surviving happily on nature's own bountiful fare, have an enormous capacity for healing – far superior to we humans.

A documentary on television not so long ago showed a camera team following a family of monkeys. The team had followed them that long that they gave the monkeys names and they were all easily identifiable.

On one occasion, one of the monkeys injured himself, resulting in a broken leg. The television crew were fearful for its survival as it limped along behind the rest of the troop. They feared that, when they came back to film again, that monkey would have died.

Two weeks later, when they returned to resume filming, they were astonished to see the animal that had the broken limb bouncing around in full flight, playing happily with his companions. Such is the astonishing rate of repair in wild nature when allowed to take its own course, without interference by outsiders.

The power to heal our bodies is within all of us. We are brought up to revere doctors and instinctively seek them when our health is in trouble. But you have to realise that doctors, nurses, hospitals, drugs, and all they entail, are completely *unnatural*. In primitive times, there were no doctors. And in wild nature today, there are no doctors, or vets. And, in wild nature, disease is virtually unknown.

But, whilst surgeons can carry out wonderful work, in separating conjoined twins or repairing serious injury after an accident, most of the time our bodies can heal themselves, if we permit any healing to take its natural course.

Any illness you may experience will doubtless be addressed with medication from your doctor. And, whilst such medication may provide temporary, and welcome, relief, that relief may come at an additional cost to your health by its toxic presence within your body.

One of the first things medical students are taught is that all drugs are toxic; it is all a matter of degree. So, that drug you are taking for your headache may well paralyse the area that is causing trouble, but at the same time adding poison to your system, especially if the drugs are continually prescribed in a cumulative fashion, as drugs tend to be given. They can have a long-term build-up effect that no-one can truly measure.

And when you are taking – as many older people do – a combination of drugs every day, then there can also be a crossover toxic effect that drug companies simply have not tested for. And any subsequent symptoms you may eventually get after being on prescription drugs for a while may be the result of the combined toxic effect on your system of the cocktail of drugs you are taking.

And do not expect your family doctor to accept this. A colleague's relative was on a cocktail of such drugs for numerous conditions, and, despite my trying to get her to see sense, she was frightened to come off any of them for fear of her symptoms becoming worse (which can be the case, so you should never cease drugs unless monitored by your family doctor).

However, she did get up enough courage to ask her doctor if, indeed, the many pills she was being prescribed could be part of her continuing poor health. The doctor merely went through the tablets, one by one, explaining that this one was for that symptom, and this other one was for another symptom, and so on – justifying the prescribing of all of them. His independent thinking that perhaps, just perhaps, the entire cocktail might be responsible for the patient's continuing health problems – just didn't seem to materialise.

The long-term sufferer from a condition such as arthritis may be given medication for years. All the time the symptoms might ease up on such drug-taking, but, when they wear off, the arthritis is still there. There has been no cure. It is the same with over a hundred chronic conditions – doctors have no cure and most certainly do not know the *cause* of most of them. As Dr Shelton would always remind his students: to cure a disease you must remove the cause. Once you find the cause, and remove it, a cure can be achieved.

Doctors are trained simply to diagnose and prescribe help for the condition, to alleviate the suffering. They are not taught to find and produce a cure.

I am not alone in believing that the future of the world's health lies in nutritional medicine, not in the dispensing of drugs. The medical profession might be able to "cure" a diseased kidney by removing it from the body, but is that really a cure? They may be able to "cure" breast cancer by slicing off the breast of the patient, but is that really a *cure*? It is no better than cutting someone's head off to cure a headache, or amputating someone's foot because he has a painful toe.

Doctors give little attention to the cause of illnesses, but concentrate all their efforts on finding an appropriate pharmaceutical product which will go only some way to providing temporary relief.

The logic in taking someone who has a health problem and, without finding or removing the cause of that problem, adding to that person's compromised system some toxic pharmaceutical products, often over many years, simply is *not* good science!

This state of affairs, prevalent in most countries, is especially worrying because drugs are *not* tested on humans over the long term (months or years), contrary to popular belief. We become long-term guinea pigs when the drug is passed as "safe" and approved for sale to the public.

The number of drugs subsequently recalled after being declared safe is testament to how ineffective, how inefficient, how completely unreliable, their testing is.

Eminent scientists and doctors from around the world, including double Nobel Prize winner, the late Linus Pauling, have become disillusioned with drugs and their toxic consequences.

The wonderful healing ability that we all have is given little leeway to perform its undoubted miracles in our modern society. We rely on the doctor or hospital to put right our many illnesses, when, more often than not, if the condition is left to run its course, it will heal of its own accord.

The body, having sustained and dealt with the "attack", will be all the stronger for it. Think, for example, of the "immunity" one dose of an infection such as measles can confer on a patient, if the condition is allowed to run its course, unimpeded by drugs.

Nature is the master healer – if given the chance. Too often fear takes over and the unnatural process of taking a chemical drug in order to cure kicks in, overwhelming common sense.

Therefore, if poor nutritional status was at the back of the original illness, now there is a further complication – toxic drugs being put into the body, *without* any change in the wrong diet that was responsible in the first place.

Whilst our family doctor will recognise that all healing will take place within the body, by the body, he will not have been trained on how to *maximise* or strengthen that healing ability.

The true extent of Nature's healing powers is there for all to see – if we only look. The small cut, the tiny graze, they all heal, and we don't even pay attention to them. But bigger, more ominous diseases can also be turned around from a seemingly terminal prognosis to total health. Often, conditions that doctors will dismiss as being "inoperable" or "terminal" can be removed and health restored to the patient.

If you consider that referring to "Nature Cure" sounds dated and smacks of Austrian health clinics of fifty or a hundred years ago, you have to realise that you cannot get much more old fashioned than Nature – nor more powerful.

Rip yourself away from the modern way of thinking, that every ill has a pill, and peer into the wonderful healing powers of Mother Nature that she is, or can be, capable of.

Let us look at an example of Nature performing her unseen, but absolutely beautifully-orchestrated miracle of healing. Let us see how a broken leg repairs itself.

The following is from *How Nature Heals* (Emmet Densmore, 1892):

"If the bone of a man or any animal be broken, and the parts replaced, the presiding and guiding force of the animal economy – call it Nature or what you will – at once deposits a liquid substance over the entire surface of the bone, a short distance in opposite directions from the fracture. This liquid soon hardens into a bone-like substance and becomes a ring firmly attached to each section of the broken bone, and for a time affords the chief support whereby the damaged limb can be used. In due time the ends of the bone – which, perhaps, had been entirely severed – become united.

Nature establishes a circulation through its parts, whereby each part is again nourished; and the limb, having its broken bone reunited, is able to support the weight of the body without calling upon the strength of the bone ring which had been temporarily built around the fractured bone.

What happens? Nature, finding no doubt that all needless supports are a damage, proceeds to soften and absorb this bone ring until it is all removed, except a slight portion for an eighth or a quarter of an inch about the point of fracture.

A similar and more familiar phenomenon is seen whenever and wherever the skin is broken; at once there is an exudation of blood; this coagulates upon exposure to the air, and forms an excellent airtight protection (a scab) to the injured part, which remains for a longer or shorter period, as may be needed, and when Nature has formed a new skin underneath, and the scab is no longer required, Nature proceeds to undermine and separate it; and while as long as it was needed it was firmly attached, as soon as it is no longer required, it falls off of its own weight.

Similarly, a sliver becomes imbedded in the flesh – a frequent accident. If a surgeon is at hand and removes it, well and good – Nature soon repairs the damage. If a surgeon is not at hand and the sliver is thus permitted to remain, Nature at once sets about a bit of fascinating engineering. First there is pain and inflammation; then follows a formation of pus; this in due time breaks down the tissues immediately surrounding the sliver, especially toward the surface of the limb. The pus increases, breaks through, runs out, and sooner or later carries the sliver with it."[32]

No surgeon needed!

You only need look at animals in the wild to witness Nature working unimpeded, when she is not being hampered in her efforts by medications or highly poisonous chemical preparations. The knitting of bones in wild animals occurs all the time, without splints or nurses or doctors. It is easy to understand how man can, with medical assistance from a hospital outpatient department, recover fully from a broken leg. It is less easy to grasp how such healing can be achieved in a dumb animal in the forest or jungle, without such help. But such healing in the wild happens all the time.

In his book *The Sex Life of Wild Animals*, Eugene Burns provides us with the following brief account of the healing of broken bones in the wild.

"One study on mammalian bone healing in the wild is truly amazing. Of ninety-five opossum skeletons taken at random near Lawrence, Kansas, thirty-nine had broken bones which had healed perfectly. Many had survived broken ribs and shoulders, some of these sustained, presumably, in competitive male fighting. One opossum had recovered from a total of two broken shoulders, eleven broken ribs (two of which had been broken twice) and a badly damaged vertebral column!

Certainly many of these injuries sustained by the opossum might have finished off heavier creatures. The recuperative power of a wild creature is enormous; broken legs slough off their decayed flesh and grow whole again, parasite-riddled organs heal, old-rotted tissues renew fresh and clean."

That does destroy the usual argument that if you don't put a broken limb into a splint, it will heal awkwardly, imprecisely, or unevenly. Eugene Burns states that the broken bones healed perfectly. We are so used to doctors tending our wounds that we defend our own methods of repair against what might seem primitive. But primitive is Nature, and nothing matches Nature in her ability to heal.

Examples of such repairs have been collected from every animal species in wild nature. The animals' wounds heal and their broken bones knit without the "advantage" of a surgeon or physician to set their broken bones or give them an anti-tetanus injection. They do not receive an anti-rabies vaccine, their wounds are not dressed or treated with antiseptics, and no-one gives them antibiotics.

Healing is a continuous process in Nature. She strives continually to attain full health. However, our daily artificial diets impede seriously the ability of the body to achieve full healing under every circumstance.

We are healed all the time of minor injuries, to which we give no conscious attention. The many little scratches, cuts, bruises, twists and tears which we receive almost daily, but which are so insignificant that we do nothing about them, are quickly healed.

Sometimes the process is so rapid that a small injury of this kind is healed completely overnight. We mash a finger with a hammer, the tissues are bruised and mangled. In a day or two the finger is healed and the incident is forgotten, although we have applied no supposed treatment. The healing of more serious injuries is accomplished with the same powers and processes by which these minor injuries are healed; the chief difference being that it takes more time.

Whilst animals in the wild, as stated by Eugene Burns, have recuperative powers that are "enormous", you have to recognise that animals in the wild do not eat their foods out of packets and tins, which may be heated. They do not eat highly cooked and processed foods that have been chemically sprayed, heated, and adulterated in order to prolong their shelf lives. Their diet is as Nature intended – natural and raw. They also do not consume toxic chemicals in the form of drugs as part of their diet whenever they may fall ill, or continue to take them for months or years on end. The wild animal is free from such an unnatural assault on its system.

Man's recuperative powers could be "enormous" if he were to follow the example of animals and allow Nature to cure and not further burden his already-ill body with impediments to recovery, such as drugs.

Drugs give the appearance of healing because they appear to remove a headache or other pain, if we suffer such distress. But if the pain comes back after the drug does its work, these drugs become less and less capable of handling the problem, until eventually they do no good at all.

Yet the doctor, aware that they worked once, will often prescribe drugs for months, even years on end. All the time, residues of these drugs can accumulate in the body and cause unnoticed harm. All drugs are not automatically dispelled from the body, as you might be advised. Even those which are eliminated may well have contributed to some damage, somewhere in the system, before leaving the body.

And the further fact that one drug can lead to another is well known.

It could be called the slippery slope of pharmaceuticals: once you start taking one drug, you'll quickly need another. Researchers have outlined the familiar pattern by reviewing the drug-taking profile of the typical arthritis sufferer, who takes an NSAID for the inflammation, then a proton pump inhibitor to stop stomach damage the NSAID might cause – and the combination of the two harms the small intestine … and so another drug is needed.

The study is the first to recognise that the combination of the two drugs causes damage to the small intestine – and that is a far harder problem to resolve than any harm the NSAID might do to the large intestine.

The combination is typical in the arthritis sufferer, say researchers from the Farncombe Family Digestive Health Research Institute. The arthritis sufferer takes an NSAID – such as aspirin – to reduce inflammation and control joint pain. But the patient knows that NSAIDs cause stomach bleeding and ulcers – so he also takes a proton pump inhibitor to reduce stomach acid, and so lower the NSAID's risks.

But the chemical cocktail of the two drugs damages the small intestine, which suggests yet another drug.[33]

A drug may "remove" a headache, but it does not remove the cause. The chances are that, if you maintain the cause of that headache – whatever that cause may be, whether it be bad diet, the inhalation of a toxic fume, or whatever – the headache will return. Of course, if it was a one-off exposure to some chemical inhalant, say, then the headache could well go away of its own accord.

Your aim is to remove the cause and that is where nutritional medicine and naturopathy can provide an answer that your doctor may not. Those of us who practise these modalities look at the patient's diet and lifestyle and attempt to adjust them accordingly, to be more in tune with natural living. That often addresses and removes the *cause* of many illnesses, which approach is something not provided by your "normal" doctor. We seek to embrace the power of Nature's healing abilities; we seek to harness this massive power, not impede it.

Doctors are unaccustomed to witnessing Nature's healing powers when at her most powerful. What they do witness, instead, is a milder form of healing – which can often still do the required job – but it can take longer and sometimes be less complete.

As stated earlier, most drugs have a short, temporary effect on symptoms, and then they wear off. The patient eventually needs to take more and more to experience the same relief, or the relief the medication *once* achieved. Eventually, however, the effectiveness the drug once displayed disappears, and the taking of the medication simply becomes a habit. Despite the drug's effects waning dramatically, it will still be prescribed, often for years. What such long-term, daily poisoning does to the system is absolutely anyone's guess, but the arrival of new symptoms as a result of this heavy load of medication is a common feature of such treatment. For these new symptoms, further drugs may also be prescribed, which can be responsible for yet further, new symptoms, and so this farcical circumstance will often go on – the familiar "repeat prescription" scenario.

I remember only too well, as a boy, visiting my great-uncle, who was almost 80, each night after his wife died. As he then lived alone and had many symptoms of ill health to contend with, I had to ensure he was safe and didn't require anything. The number of pill bottles he had to sift through each night in order to complete his nightly drug-taking regimen was, even to a boy, mind boggling.

Despite the mass of drugs which his doctor instructed him to take, his symptoms were still with him, and they just worsened. He never got better. It greatly saddens me now to know what I might have been able to do for him, were I to know then what I know now. These drugs did *nothing* to restore health to my great-uncle's body. Drugs do *nothing* to restore health to *anybody's* body!

How many households, up and down the land, in this country and throughout the world, take such similar medications in the belief that these drugs will *cure* their symptoms? It is unthinkable the suffering that must go on in families – in trusting families across the globe. As has been said before in this book by a disillusioned medical doctor, the system of medicine in our modern world is one of self-deception, nothing less.

Many recoveries from ill health have been achieved by the simple expedient of removing all drugs from the patient's bedside.

I recall that Liz Taylor, the actress, once remarked that she was able to get out of her wheelchair for the first time for years once she decided to stop her growing list of medications.

And in a nursing home magazine in the U.K., I remember a story of a nursing home nurse/manager in the south of England who took the brave step of arranging for many of the patients to have their medication reduced, and, in some cases, stopped completely.

The nurse was surprised indeed when, a few days later, one of the chair-bound patients got up unaided and walked over to the front door. That was the first time that the nurse had ever seen that patient walk unaided.

There is more than enough evidence to show that drugs, despite being declared safe for your doctor to prescribe, can cause considerable harm – even death.

Dr Vernon Coleman, a medical doctor, writing in the *Journal of Alternative and Complementary Medicine* in July 1994, stated that it was estimated that over *one million* patients are in hospital beds in the U.K. as a *direct* result of iatrogenesis – damage caused by prescribed drug-taking.

Dr Herbert Shelton recalls an autopsy which was performed on a three-year-old girl in San Antonio, Texas. The child had been taken to the hospital the evening before and found to be dead on arrival. According to the father, the child was given a "dose of medicine" on the first morning for the treatment "of a cold".

During the day she became violently ill. When he returned home in the evening, the child collapsed and was dead before he could get her to the hospital.

Children, Shelton observed, do not die of colds. They do not sicken in the morning and die suddenly in the evening of the same day of a cold.

Whatever the autopsy finding may have been, we can be sure that this child died of the "cure". Whether she received the "wrong" medicine or an overdose of the "right" medicine, she died of drug poisoning. The violent illness that developed after the "remedy" was administered was the violent efforts of the little organism to rid itself of the poison.

Shelton explained: each and every one of us should realise that the only drugs in all the chemists in the land that are properly labelled are those bearing the skull and crossbones. There is no such thing as a non-poisonous drug. Some are of greater virulence than others, but all are poisonous.

Shelton recalls in his own words, in his *Hygienic Review* of April 1968, the following story which pays tribute to the power of the human organism's healing efforts when allowed to do so without interference.

"My baby is dying." These plaintive words of a despairing mother came to me over the telephone in the early morning one day in the winter of 1927 or 1928. (My records have been destroyed and an exact date is not possible.) She explained the baby was on medication and was becoming worse.

I was living in New York at the time and was on the staff of the Macfadden publications, writing for Physical Culture and other publications of that organization. I had a daily column in the New York Graphic and feature articles in the magazine section of the Graphic on occasion. The woman identified herself as Mrs Marvin Hall of Nyack, New York. I did not know Mrs Hall and she did not know me. She had been reading my articles in the Graphic and appealed to me in her distress.

I asked her: "How do you know that your baby is dying, Mrs Hall?" She replied: "My baby has pneumonia and a consultation of four doctors has just rendered this verdict. They say there is nothing more that they can do, that the baby will die."

I said to Mrs Hall: "Let's fool them!" She replied: "That is exactly what I want to do. I want my baby to live."

I said: "Mrs Hall, listen carefully and follow these instructions exactly. Go to the bedside of your baby and sweep all that mass of drugs on the table by its bed into the waste basket and see that the baby does not get another dose of drugs. Open the window and let some fresh air into the room. Keep the baby warm. Give it no food. Give it water according to thirst. Report to me tomorrow morning."

Each morning for the next few mornings, Mrs Hall called me on the telephone and reported the daily progress of her baby. The progress was much faster than we could have hoped for and the baby's recovery was soon complete. About 20 years passed and Madelyn Hall – the baby's name – now grown into a lovely young lady, was married."

The above is a vivid – and frightening – description of the limitations doctors work under. Although that was nearly one hundred years ago, the same situation will still arise today, all too regularly.

Shelton was keen to state that very often the "complications" that result in the death of someone have actually been caused by the toxic medications given to the patient and they have died from the unknown effects of the drug on that particular patient's system, and not the original condition. Although, in such a case, you can rest assured that the cause of death on the death certificate won't point to any drug administered as being responsible.

However, I should once again warn the reader that no steps should be taken to reduce or cease medication without the monitoring – and approval – of your doctor.

14.

Breast Cancer Cured in 1929
Using Raw, Natural Food

There appeared in *Nature's Way Monthly* (England), back in January 1929, the following report of recovery from a case of cancer and the crises through which the patient passed in her progress towards recovery. Flare-ups, or crises, in the form of symptoms getting worse and even new symptoms appearing are a peculiar phenomenon in Nature Cure recovery. This story highlights just that very point.

This account was reproduced in April 1929's edition of *How to Live*:

"Yes, you would marvel were you to investigate a case in a Devonshire village – a case dismissed as beyond the power of surgery nearly six months ago. In July last year, the sufferer adopted the non-medical treatment advocated in the Nature's Way publications: this is a last hope, and rather a forlorn one. The left breast was then of enormous size, and of a deep purple hue; the right breast was in a stage of inflammation, while lumps were developing about the neck and arms. The malady continued to develop, and the brave soul even gained courage while she watched the progress of her affliction, trusting to Nature's process of purification.

The manifestation of that process has been indeed a revelation. By the effort of Nature to throw out the poisons in this woman's blood, through the simple means of a pure dietary, the sufferer's skin became overlaid with patches of knotted flakes, terrible to see, from the head to the knees; the eyes and ears exuded matter, and clusters of warts sprouted over the arms and shoulders.

The body of this tormented creature steamed perspiration in its agony at the crisis! Humanly speaking, she was doomed, and she is one in a hundred thousand to have clung to the remotest hope of rescue, since she had arrived at such a pass without the succour which is supposed to come from morphia and other medical methods.

The culmination came and went, and, as one who stood in the presence of this case, as the Editor of this Journal stood but a few hours since, was brought face to face with a phenomenon of astounding significance. The woman has risen from her bed, her breast is shrunk to its normal size, new pinkish skin replaces the falling encrusted patches, glandular swelling and scattered lumps have subsided, the warts are disappearing as mysteriously as they came, and there is an absence of that dreadful odour so characteristic of malignancy.

This instance of Nature's rebuilding power is one which should permit of doubt or denial in the light of further progress towards recovery. This message to you concerns an illustration of Nature's method of conflict with disease, and therein is an opportunity offered to scientific research to witness, and to learn from the issue of the struggle.

And it should be added that this victim of lifelong folly had suffered from constipation from infancy, she received the ministrations of twenty-seven practitioners, she followed the constant habit of taking aperients, she had lain as a patient in four hospitals, and for the past twelve years had known no relief from stomach troubles. Yet medical journals, new, as well as otherwise, adjure medical consultation at the earliest signs of the affliction – such signs as twenty-seven members of the profession had failed to note, or act upon in this woman's increasing and evident distress.

But let us regard a brief statement of the facts presented by the experience of this particular sufferer. In July last year, the disease had already gained so grave a hold upon her system that a well-known surgeon refused to operate. Clinging to the last straw, as it were, she asked him if he thought diet would help her, as she had read in a local paper that simple feeding was suggested, by certain writers, as the remedy for nearly all disorders, even including cancer.

He answered that dieting would not be a bit of good, but that radium might relieve the pain, and he intimated that recovery was impossible.

Left to her own resources, the woman dared to trust a course that had been dismissed as futile. She fed on fruit and salads almost entirely, she poulticed the wounds with apple pulp, and rubbed oil and fruit juice over the parts that were inflamed and hard. She persevered in the way on which she had embarked, notwithstanding that appearances, for some time, gave little prospect of any improvement in her condition.

Herein lies the secret of Nature's dealings with disease; there can be no hurrying. The bad works of many years, as in her case, could not be undone within a month. The whole of her frame required cleansing; indeed, it needed reconstruction. She was a complete pollution.

Therefore, in the process of eliminating the accumulated waste, and in repairing the disorganised structure, the state of congestion was increased externally, so that, on seeing it, one would have said she was worse, for all her heroic patience.

How could surgery – or its whilom competitor, radium – have eradicated conditions which saturated this woman's body, through the vitiated blood stream? There are cases of cancer, as well as other disorders, due to the one root cause, in which bones have become so rotten as to fracture spontaneously.

Is it possible for the knife, or any similar expedient, to cut out, or incinerate, an all-embracing evidence of corruption?

Before us lies a letter from one who, having a slight swelling of the breast, has been advised an operation as a prevention of cancer, notwithstanding that the symptoms of her case show no indications of her malady! Surely, if such a persuasion has reason in it, our bodies should be dismembered as a precaution against the chances of disease in any part of us! This is indeed anticipation by barbarity, a resource too horrible to be believed of those to whom we attribute intelligence and sympathy.

In this instance, then, of which we have personal knowledge, the crisis was not reached until the last day of November, when, judging by appearances, cancer and not Nature had sealed the sufferer's doom. How could the raging torment have been comprehended as the portent of a contrary result? What desperate means could one adopt to meet such desperate exigencies?

Nothing could humanly avail but to leave Nature alone to her mysterious purpose; and so they wore on, whilst those who saw it stood dumbfounded at the spectacle.

By the following day the conflict had been fought. The hours of agony were followed by a rapid decrease of congestion, and with it was shown a revelation of Nature's reconstructive power, in the appearance of new wholesome skin beneath the thick, dry burnt-up scales of waste that fell from the sufferer's arms and shoulders, chest, and back.

This phenomenon should have been witnessed by those who declare that there are no means of coping with cancer but by methods of mutilation; and the endurance of this woman – her astounding courage, with the amazing vitality given to her for her defence – can be considered by any who may be sufficiently interested in her case to apply to the Editor of this journal for photographic records which were taken within a fortnight of the crisis referred to."

Dr Shelton said of cancer: "Cancer can never develop in a healthy organ. It would be impossible for cancer to develop in a perfect healthy body. It is always an evolution out of prior diseased states, whether one is aware of it or not."

Shelton also made the following relevant remarks on the treatment of disease in general: "We can no more cure disease than we can heal a wound or knit a broken bone. Nature does all the curing that is ever done. She usually succeeds in spite of crucifying treatment. She succeeded in the days of heroic dosage. She succeeded in the days of the witch broth and incantation. She succeeds in these days of 'progress'. And it is fortunate for man that nature does cure, else he would surely have become extinct."

15.

The Gerson Cancer Therapy

This famous dietary therapy has produced astonishing recoveries from many common, but debilitating, health problems. It is not an entirely raw diet, but it has a large raw content, mainly of salads and juices.

There is a cooked element to the therapy – hot soup and potatoes are allowed – this making it all the more acceptable to our cooked-food palates.

Whilst it is not entirely raw, its large raw content is sufficient to restore health to many people suffering from a wide range of symptom complexes. The therapy was brought to the American shores in the 1930s by Max Gerson, a German doctor.

To this day it is a thorn in the side of the American medical establishment, who refuse to accept that by improving the health of the patient with a superior diet to which they already eat, the body can recover from a variety of illnesses, including cancers.

The fact that a similar dietary treatment is recognised in Holland – the Moerman Diet – does not seem to convince those in charge of health in America that there really is another way to treat cancer. And more successfully than the present American medical paradigm of toxic drugs.

Beata Bishop, a former BBC researcher from London, recovered from terminal cancer by following the diet; now she travels around Europe lecturing on the therapy. Beata wrote a book on her experience, entitled *A Time to Heal,*[34] and Dr Gerson's daughter, Charlotte, and grandson, Howard, both lecture throughout the United States and Canada on the therapy.

Dr Max Gerson, M.D., was born in 1881 in Wongrowitz, Germany. He attended the universities of Breslau, Wuerzburg, Berlin, and Freiburg. He was director of a special department of tuberculosis at the Munich

University Hospital under the sponsorship of Dr Ferdinand Sauerbruch, a world famous thoracic surgeon and tuberculosis authority.

As a young German medical student, Gerson suffered from severe migraine headaches. He had been told that they were untreatable and that he would have to learn to live with them. But Gerson experimented with his diet in an effort to find relief from the headaches which kept him in bed for days at a time.

To his joy, Gerson found that by restricting his diet, by avoiding salt, fats, pickled and smoked foods, and by eating fresh fruits and vegetables, he could control them. Soon, he was sharing this new "migraine diet" with his patients.

One of Gerson's patients insisted that the migraine diet had cured his skin tuberculosis. Gerson listened, carefully weighing up the possibility that the diet might somehow be enhancing immunity. He decided that it might be true and set out to validate it. In the process, his work came to the attention of Sauerbruch. A new era in medicine was born.

In 1929, Sauerbruch announced Gerson's dietary therapy as a *cure* for skin TB, publishing simultaneously in a dozen of the world's leading peer-reviewed scientific journals. Sauerbruch told of a clinical trial of Gerson's dietary treatment in which 446 out of 450 TB patients achieved lasting cures (also mentioned in Sauerbruch's autobiography, *Master Surgeon*). Gerson lectured in the principal cities of Europe until the pre-war political climate forced him to emigrate to America in 1933.

During this time, Gerson attracted the friendship of Nobel Prize winner Albert Schweitzer, M.D., by curing his wife Helena Schweitzer of lung tuberculosis after she had failed to respond to all conventional managements.

1934 saw the publication of *Diet Therapy for Lung Tuberculosis* (pub. Franz Deuticke, Leipzig and Vienna), in which Mrs Schweitzer's recovery is documented as case number 45.

Gerson and Schweitzer remained friends for life and maintained regular correspondence. Schweitzer followed Gerson's progress as the diet therapy was applied successfully to a wide variety of pathologies, including heart and kidney failure, and finally cancer. Schweitzer's own adult-onset diabetes responded to Gerson's dietary treatment.

In 1938, Gerson demonstrated recovered cancer patients before the Pepper-Neely Congressional Sub-Committee, during hearings on S.1875, a bill to authorise the American President to wage war on cancer. Although only a few peer-reviewed journals were receptive to his revolutionary ideas, Gerson continued to publish in the U.S. and abroad.

In 1958, after 30 years of clinical experimentation, Gerson published *A Cancer Therapy: Results of Fifty Cases.*[35] This medical monograph details the theories, the treatment, and the results achieved by a great physician. A more recent version has been published by his daughter, Charlotte Gerson, along with Morton Walker, entitled *The Gerson Therapy: The Proven Nutritional Program for Cancer and Other Illnesses.*[36]

Gerson died in 1959. He was eulogised by Albert Schweitzer:

"I see in him one of the most eminent geniuses in the history of medicine. Many of his basic ideas have been adopted without having his name connected with them. Yet he has achieved more than seemed possible under adverse conditions. He leaves a legacy which commands attention and which will assure him his due place. Those whom he cured will now attest to the truth of his ideas."

There are thousands of case histories of recovered patients at the Gerson Institute in California. Because treating cancer with nutrition was declared a criminal offence in America, the Gerson doctors moved to a clinic in Mexico, where acceptance of "alternative" methods of treatment exists.

The Gerson therapy strengthens a patient's immune system, which is what you would need to recover from illness, whilst the conventional method of treatment for cancer – chemotherapy – not only destroys the patient's immune system, but has an astonishingly low success rate.

Just some examples of the thousands of recoveries from cancer using the Gerson therapy are given here:

****

Jacquie Davison (who recounted her full story in the book *Cancer Winner*) had tumours all over her head, neck, abdomen, diaphragm, arms and legs. Her abdomen bloated to 30 lbs. Her doctor gave her no more than three weeks to live and she was advised her death would be swift and certain. She gave away most of her possessions and made her own funeral dress.

Her family encouraged her on to the Gerson therapy. She had many "healing crises", but made a full recovery. Her book was recently reprinted.

****

The story of Helga Braun is extraordinary and extremely rare in cases of breast cancer treated by orthodox means. When she was 32 years old, she didn-t feel well and detected a nodule in her breast. She went to her doctor, who ordered a mammogram, which "showed nothing". He sent her home, suggesting she was a hypochondriac. However, still not feeling well, she felt deep down that something was definitely wrong. She once more visited her doctor and again was told that she was just imagining things and that there was nothing wrong with her. Finally, on her third visit, she insisted that the doctor do a thorough study of the lump which was still in her breast. When he finally agreed and did a biopsy, the tissue turned out to be positive for "medullary carcinoma".

Subsequently, her surgeon, Dr John Baldwin, at the Community Hospital in Monterey, California, did a partial mastectomy in 1979. This was followed by six weeks of "standard" radiation.

But Helga had a friend who suggested that she change her diet and lifestyle and gave her information about the Gerson therapy. She followed the programme carefully for one year and felt much better. She continued to follow the nutritional care that had achieved so much and was in good health thirty years after her surgery and radiation.

****

In July 2005, at the age of 68, Joyce Forsythe found an "enormous mass" in her abdomen. In her own words: "PET and CT scans showed my spleen had grown to the size of a football. I had my spleen removed and a biopsy showed a diagnosis of stage IV mantle cell, non-Hodgkin's lymphoma. My oncologist at Dana Farber recommended a cocktail of four different chemotherapy drugs, including a trial drug, to be infused weekly into a Mediport surgically implanted in my upper chest for six months. He hoped these drugs would put my cancer into remission for a couple of years. If the cancer came back, different chemotherapeutic drugs would be needed the next time around, because the same drugs wouldn't work a second time.

"I learned about Dr Max Gerson's therapy 30 years earlier when we lived outside of New York City, where he used to have his office. As a long-time subscriber to the Gerson newsletter, I always planned, if ever I were to get cancer, to immediately start the Gerson. I turned down the chemotherapy and told my oncologist that I would do Max Gerson's holistic cancer therapy instead. He reminded me that my cancer was stage IV and, while nutrition wouldn't hurt, it wouldn't help. I had read Dr Gerson's book and the many patient cases in the newsletters over the years, so the oncologist's warnings were no deterrent for me.

"Now retired, my husband Pete and I felt up to the task of rebuilding my body with hourly fresh vegetable juices and all that is required by the therapy. Along with the hard work involved, there were lots of chuckles, like when Pete reported to me that the grocery clerk, ringing up a 20-pound bag of carrots, commented, 'I know, you have a horse'.

"We were both overjoyed as my lab results began showing the healing taking place.

"I had not been on the Gerson therapy long when I took my latest lab reports with me to an appointment with my oncologist at Dana Farber.

"I asked for the name of an oncologist in Florida who could oversee my case for the next six months while we were away. My oncologist took a look at the lab results and exclaimed, 'These are absolutely fantastic!' then added, 'I don't think you'll need an oncologist while you're gone.' I soon received a letter from him saying I should keep doing whatever I was doing, adding that the chemotherapy would not have cured my cancer. Although the lymphoma specialist at Dana Farber Cancer Institute in Boston was in charge of my case, CT scans, blood tests and cancer marker tests were done at our local cancer centre and I met regularly with my local oncologist, for interpretation of the results. The local oncologist told me at the end of five years that there was no need for me to keep coming to see her; however, she said she didn't want to lose touch with my case.

"She said she thinks of me often as she prescribes for others the drugs that had been recommended for me. She doubts that I would be so healthy today if I had taken the chemo offered. She asked if I would be willing to send her a copy of the annual lab results ordered by my internist for my future physicals. She would look over them and then we could talk on the phone, or, better yet, she'd prefer that I meet with her in person without charging for the appointments. I told her I'd welcome that. 'One last thing,' she added. 'Make one last appointment with your oncologist at Dana Farber and share with him the details of your case. When you leave, give him a bill.' We chuckled. 'Seriously,' she said, 'we doctors need to know about your success.'

"The following week, I went to my internist for my annual physical. After the exam, she commented, 'You could be a poster girl for how a woman of 73 should be eating.' This same internist wrote in my annual report, 'Mrs Forsythe has cured her own cancer following Gerson therapy to the "T".' "

* * * * * * * * * * * * * * * *

John Kennedy was born in 1938. At the end of the 1970s, he noted irregular rectal bleeding, dark in colour. He went to see his doctor in El Cajon, California, who did a rectal blood test as well as a barium enema (barium is used in order to make the colon visible on an X-ray picture). John had no surgery. The physician diagnosed colon cancer that had spread, confirmed by the X-rays; and he found metastases to the liver. He told John to "get his affairs in order, make his will, and prepare his wife".

John didn't like the idea, and set off to do some research. He found some books by Carlton Fredricks. With his new ideas, he went to a health food store, where he found a "familiar" name. It was Dr Max Gerson's *A Cancer Therapy: Results of 50 Cases.* A neighbour he met at the store spoke to John about his own colon cancer, cured by the book John held in his hand, *A Cancer Therapy.*

Then John found the Gerson Institute, called and visited their office in San Diego, where he got information about the Gerson Therapy Hospital and arranged a stay there. He was treated by Dr Melendez and was put on the Gerson therapy. In one week, John had a heavy "healing reaction", after which he felt much better, "almost euphoric".

He continued the therapy at home with the K & K press type juicer. It was difficult for his handicapped wife. During this time, they moved "up north" to Mendocino County, where John had pure, uncontaminated spring water and fresh air.

In a few months, John felt much better and, after six months, he says, "I felt about normal". He stayed with the Gerson therapy for two and a half years. When he went back to his original doctor, he sent for John's records, looked at them, and said, "If you were cured of cancer, I don't know what idiot diagnosed you." John suggested the doctor look at the signature on the records; it was his own! Later, when John asked for his records at the V.A. Hospital, they had been "modified"!

****

Marge Lemly suffered from heart disease and emphysema. Later, she had a nervous breakdown, and a heart attack with sharp chest pains, and was put on oxygen. She was unable to move and had extreme breathing difficulties. Her doctors prescribed digitalis, nitroglycerine and valium.

She was offered, but refused, enderol. She lost 76 lbs in weight. She began the Gerson therapy in October 1979, regained weight and was alive and well at last contact twelve years later, in 1991.

80

****

Dr James Clark had non-healing infections, arrhythmia (abnormal heart rate) and insomnia. He suffered an ankle injury that would not heal. He had 13 operations and grafts which also would not heal.

After a year in hospital, his leg was removed below the knee. He continued to have infections, was given drugs and antibiotics, but still suffered arrhythmias, stomach distress, confusion, headaches and could not concentrate. He despaired of living and was admitted to a psychiatric hospital. He began the Gerson therapy, after which he fully recovered his health.

****

Elizabeth Birdwell suffered poor health in early life, with many problems. Her mother had been prescribed drugs during pregnancy. Multiple sclerosis was diagnosed in December 1973. Bartter's Syndrome was diagnosed. She also had confirmed hypothyroidism, hypoglycaemia, multiple allergies, early kidney failure, convulsions, profound exhaustion and muscle weakness.

She started the Gerson therapy in May 1984. There was steady improvement. She recovered fully to work as a model, attend university and get married. She was well at the last contact in 1991, seven years after starting the therapy.

****

Susan Adams had spreading melanoma (highly malignant tumour). She had moles removed from her right wrist. Malignant melanoma was confirmed by an outside hospital in January 1980. Three pathologists from the University of California agreed on the diagnosis. The tumour spread into the right axilla (armpit) and was surgically cut out. The cancer continued spreading.

She began the Gerson therapy in November 1980 and achieved complete recovery. She had a recurrence after pregnancy, but recovered again.

****

Identical twins, Mary and Martha Ormesher, were diagnosed as having a fatal disease, Takayasu's Arteritis (Pulseless Disease). It started with Mary in 1978, when she was 16. She had an infection, diarrhoea, severe headaches, pain on breathing, and extreme chest pains. Her doctor, Dr Johnson, found no blood pressure or pulse in her right arm. Takayasu's was diagnosed. This diagnosis was confirmed by an outside clinic (the Mayo Clinic) in February 1979. She was given prednisone. Dr Roland Johnson (Diplomate: American Board of Internal Medicine) said: "This is a uniformly malignant and fatal arteritis." A few months later, her twin sister Martha had the same symptoms and was similarly diagnosed.

Mary began the Gerson therapy in June 1980. Martha began in August. As well as the Gerson, they took some herbs. There was steady improvement. From a "certain" death sentence, both girls fully recovered and were active at last contact, a full 20 years later.

****

Melva Blackburn had diabetes, arthritis, Alzheimer's Disease, kidney and adrenal disease, Cushing's Syndrome, and other symptoms. She had medical problems from 1944 onwards and was treated till 1979. She was given drugs for her heart (coronary artery) disease, and drugs to treat her diabetes (from 1965). She had poor control of her legs and feet, and suffered from Cushing's Syndrome (adrenal disease, obesity, fatigue, weakness, osteoporosis, oedema, infections), pneumonia twice a year, an enlarged liver, arthritis in all joints, anxiety, ataxia (unsteady gait), confusion, asphasia (speech difficulty). Alzheimer's was diagnosed. She had been on drugs for many years and had many operations for her problems. She began the Gerson therapy in October 1979 and rapidly recovered. All diseases disappeared without any drugs. She astounded her doctors and remains active and well, aged 83 at last contact.

****

Marilyn Dent had 11 operations in 11 years. She suffered from migraines, tachycardia, hypoglycaemia and mental illness. She had a hysterectomy and various exploratory operations. Surgery injured the sciatic nerve, giving her constant severe pain and sharp intermittent pain from head to feet. She was given many drugs for her various symptoms, suffered a nervous breakdown, and was admitted to a psychiatric ward.

She began the Gerson therapy in October 1977 and showed rapid improvement. She came off all drugs, and was restored to good health, living a normal life.

****

David Nelson (son of Bill Nelson, below) was diagnosed as having "hopeless" astrocytoma brain cancer in January 1986. He had a grand mal seizure. Surgery removed 50% of the tumour, which was described as lemon-sized with many "crabgrass roots" into the brain remaining. A biopsy confirmed astrocytoma (brain tumour), and doctors gave him between 2 and 12 months to live. He began the Gerson therapy in April 1986. Four MRI scans in 3 years showed reduction and then complete disappearance of the tumour.

****

Bill Nelson (father of David, above) suffered from Candida (yeast infection) and was prone to chemical sensitivity. After a restaurant meal in 1977, he had a hard time breathing. He was given drugs without any diagnosis. In 1978, he had the first of five sinus operations. These didn't help. He couldn't breathe and was given more drugs, including antibiotics. He had white fungus spots on the mouth and private parts and probably had yeast infection in the lungs. 60mg cortisone daily gave no relief. He couldn't sleep. He was on continuous oxygen. He began the Gerson therapy in 1986, with immediate improvement. Completely recovered, he built a house and remained well.

****

Alexandra Lennox had breast cancer biopsied in 1984, with nodules on breast and liver, plus medically diagnosed herpes simplex, Epstein-Barr, hypoglycaemia, chronic fatigue syndrome, histo-plasmosis (virus from birds), and severe depression. She began the Gerson therapy in May 1984. Today she is alive, healthy, active and full of life. Tests show she is completely free of breast cancer. She has now published her book, *Alive and Cancer Free*. She is proud to state that, "The fresh organic foods and juices of the Gerson therapy saved my life!"

****

Bill Goerdes, who passed away at nearly 100, was diagnosed with severe rheumatoid arthritis and bleeding stomach ulcers in 1941. New York Presbyterian Medical Centre X-rays showed his spine fused top to bottom with rheumatoid arthritis. He was offered no hope. He began Gerson therapy with Dr Gerson in October 1941, and his ulcers were gone in six weeks. He was able to return to light work in seven and a half months and commenced heavier duties in 14 months. Completely restored to health by the therapy, he was well and active for almost 60 years. (It is interesting to note that Charlotte Gerson confirmed to me that Bill, whose spine was "fused top to bottom", had his "bones restored and separated"!)

****

Deanna Powell had severe rheumatoid arthritis and was bedridden in 1976. She suffered constant pain and stiffness. All her joints were swollen; her elbows, knees and most fingers were bent and frozen. She had bony deformities and walked with great difficulty. She had heart palpitations, laboured breathing and was pale, anaemic and had hypoglycaemia. She was taking 15-20 aspirins daily, but still had pain and insomnia. She began the Gerson in May 1978. In six weeks the pain was gone and most lumps had started to dissolve. All problems were resolved, except a few joints which were not quite clear. She got married and had a family, experiencing a recurrence of her symptoms after pregnancy, from which she recovered. She took up water skiing and enjoys life.

****

Many doctors will state that these are only "anecdotal" stories of recovery. But the fuller details and records of these cases are kept at the Gerson Institute.

Whilst the Gerson therapy involves 13 glasses of raw, organic vegetable and fruit juices per day, as well as a large raw salad and soups (these hot soups make the diet more satisfying for many who are used to cooked foods), it is not something that modern medical science is set up to evaluate.

Their tests are geared towards drugs. They will give one group of patients a placebo, and another group the real drug which is being tested, to evaluate if the drug works or not.

But how could such a testing regimen work with diet? How could one group of patients get a dummy placebo pill and the other group the real therapy – a huge diet full of salads and juices – without each group knowing what they were taking?

Even if medical science *wanted* to test any dietary method (but they *don't*), that method would be futile. And certainly no real attempts to evaluate such a diet have been carried out in medicine, for fear, it has been said, of finding out they worked.

There simply is no *will* – no *desire* – by medical scientists to evaluate such a dietary approach to cancer. Because, as explained elsewhere, it would make a mockery of their billions of dollars and pounds spent on so-called "research". And, it would put a stop to the heavily-funded gravy train that give these professionals such high standards of living. If you were a cancer researcher and you found out that such a simple thing as what you ate was responsible for the disease and that by adhering to a natural diet – free from processing or refining – the illness could be reversed, would you want to hear that, which effectively could wipe out your own career?

Beata Bishop states:

"One of the bonuses of the therapy is that it heals the entire organism, not just the presenting, main, problem. In other words, it heals the patient, not the disease. This was a major discovery for Dr Gerson, as his orthodox medical training at three top German universities had taught him that any treatment only addressed a particular condition and nothing else. He was forced to abandon that principle as a young doctor when he found that his "migraine diet" also cured skin tuberculosis. It was this recognition that, given the right conditions, the body could heal itself of several illnesses. It was this recognition that led him to develop his cancer treatment. A less intensive form of the therapy can cure a wide range of chronic conditions.

My own experience confirms the validity of Dr Gerson's approach. When I embarked on the therapy, beside the spreading melanoma, I also suffered from early stage diabetes mellitus, incipient osteoarthritis and painful recurrent dental abscesses. Within three weeks at the Gerson clinic in Mexico, all three conditions simply vanished, never to return. Moreover, my surgically mutilated right leg began to grow back some flesh, a process which I watched with jaw-dropping amazement. Getting rid of the melanoma took much longer, though; the body prefers to deal with the easy bits first!

Orthodoxy rejects and often attacks it, without knowing what it is attacking. Gerson-trained doctors are few and far between. Most Gerson therapists come from the complementary, or alternative medicine field. Lack of funds prevents the setting up of controlled prospective trials; hence, peer-reviewed reports are thin on the ground. At present the world's only Gerson clinic is in Mexico, but hopefully one or two more will open up before long. Even without visiting the clinic, very many people all over the world have successfully completed the therapy, relying on Dr Gerson's classic book, A Cancer Therapy; Results of Fifty Cases, which contains precise instructions for healing at home."

The effectiveness of even a watered-down version of the Gerson protocol was demonstrated recently in a six-year clinical trial, conducted by oncologist-surgeon Dr Peter Lechner at the District Hospital in Graz, Austria. His patients did remarkably better than members of the control group, both in length of survival and quality of life.[37]

In her case history of Oxford Don Michael Gearin-Tosh's ten-year survival of multiple myeloma on the Gerson protocol, Carmen Wheatley, D.Phil.(Oxon.), shows in detail how the latest research into the cancer-fighting properties of plant compounds confirms Gerson's therapeutic choice of fruits and vegetables, and his way to deliver them to the patient intact and in the correct doses in the form of freshly made juices. Her study was peer-reviewed by four eminent oncologists.[38]

From Japan comes the testimony of Professor Yoshihiko Hoshino, Professor of Medicine at Fukushima University, Northern Japan, whose book, *How a Professor of Medicine Cured Himself of Liver-metastasised Colon Cancer with the Gerson Therapy*, is at present only available in Japanese. Starting by curing himself and 12 cancer patients on the same protocol, since 1998 he has treated over 500 more with a colleague, achieving good results and expanding the work all the time.[39]

16.

A Doctor Cures Her Own Cancer With Raw Food
by Dr Kristine Nolfi (Denmark)[40]
Originally published around 1950

Before I realised the actual importance of raw fruit and vegetable food, my attitude was exactly the same as that of other doctors – to treat the symptoms of the disease without thinking of preventing it in the first place.

It *ought* to be the duty of the medical profession in future to find means of preventing to a much higher degree than now, instead of having to cure later on.

That I, as a medical doctor, went in for an *exclusive* raw fruit and vegetable diet is due to the fact that I became ill, even seriously ill, myself. I developed cancer of the breast.

The disease had, of course, been preceded by *wrong nourishment and wrong habits* in the course of my twelve years of hospital training, when I suffered from sluggish digestion and catarrh of the stomach all the time, disorders which are still of quite common occurrence among hospital staff members. Since that time, no change in the hospital diet has taken place in Denmark in this very important domain.

On one occasion I was in a dying condition because of a bleeding gastric ulcer. This made me abandon meat and fish, and I became a vegetarian.

Later, I took to eating a good deal of raw fruits and vegetable food. In this manner my digestion became regulated, and I felt better, though not completely well. In the winter of 1940 to 1941, I was exceptionally tired and dull, but I was unable to ascertain any specific disease. At that time I did not understand what was wrong with me, but in the course of the Spring I discovered a small node in my right breast.

Tired and dull as I was, I did not pay any attention to it until, five weeks later, I discovered that the node was the size of a hen's egg. It had grown into the skin; a thing only cancer does.

As a doctor, I had seen enough to be unwilling to submit to the treatment of cancer generally employed. I consulted my good friend, Dr M. Hindhede, who dissuaded a trial microscopy. It would open up the blood streams and the cancer would spread; so I gave up.

And then I felt it as quite natural that I would have to commit to a *one hundred percent raw diet.*

I went in search of nature and lived for a time on a small island in the Kattegat, took sun baths from four to five hours daily, slept in a tent, bathed several times a day, and lived exclusively on a raw fruit and vegetable diet. Later, I introduced this habit of life at the sanatorium "Humlegaarden".

But I was still tired and continued to be so for the first two months, and during this period the node in the breast did not diminish; it remained unchanged.

But then the improvement came!

The node diminished, my strength returned. I recovered and felt better than I had done for many years.

When I had experienced good health in this manner for about a year, I tried by way of experiment (and urged to do so by Dr Hindhede) to revert to a "normal" diet supplemented by fifty percent of raw food.

But it was no good. In three or four months I began to feel a stinging pain in the breast, in the sore-like tissue which the cancer had left where it had originally adhered to the skin. *This pain increased much during the weeks that followed, and I realised that the cancer had begun to develop again.*

Once more I reverted to pure, raw food, which caused the pain to subside rapidly and the fatigue to become less pronounced.

Being a doctor, I realised that I would have to use the experience I had gained to help my sick fellow creatures. So I set up my home so that I could have four or five patients staying with me the next summer.

We took a hundred percent raw fruit and vegetable diet and all went well, but running such a clinic was not satisfactory with so few patients.

I understood that this cause would have to be advocated under quite different and larger conditions if any proofs were to be given.

On my initiative, a joint stock company was then formed which bought a property, "Humlegaarden", well suited for the purpose; it was set up as a sanatorium, where I became the chief physician. Here, we ate only raw fruit and vegetable food, patients as well as employees, and the establishment is now in its sixth year.

Now, what is the reason why a one hundred percent raw diet should exert such a beneficial effect on civilised individuals? First and foremost, because the raw food is *live food* – as it is handed to us by nature. We all know that life on earth is completely dependent on our sun. If we had no sun, the earth would be without any life, dark and icy cold. Vital force is therefore identical with sun energy!

According to Dr Hesselink, it is, however, only the plant with its widely unfolded thin green leaves that is able to catch the sunlight and to deposit it in the form of roots and tubers, fruit and seeds. We human beings, and the animals, with massive bodies, are not able to utilise it to a sufficiently high degree. Therefore, both man and beast use plants as carriers between the sun and themselves. A fresh, raw fruit and vegetable diet is sunlight nourishment!

Dr Bircher-Benner, of Zurich, realised this long ago. Dr Hesselink, from Holland, believes that it is the atoms which are the carriers of the solar energy.

Fresh, raw vegetable foods possess the highest nutritive value, and this cannot be increased or improved; anything else, such as heating, drying, storing, fermentation or preservation, will tend to reduce and destroy its value. Boiled vegetables taste of nothing, so something must be done to make them palatable. We mix many different things together; we add salt, sugar, spices and butter. We remove the germ and the husk from the wheat to use the flour for baking. We polish the rice, we refine the sugar; we remove the skin, seeds, and cores of apples and pears, we peel the potatoes and scrape the carrots. Meat, fish, eggs and cheese supply us with an enormous surplus of animal protein. We make beverages of coffee and cocoa beans, and tea, which contain stimulating poisons.

We use the grapes for wine and brandy – intoxicating poisons – which first stimulate the grey cortex of the brain, and later paralyse it. We preserve food with chemicals, such as benzoic acid, salicylic acid, nitrates, boric acid and sulphurous acid in order that it may keep well, and look attractive.

Further, we take anodynes, hypnotics, sedatives, and aperients – all strong chemical poisons – or, at any rate, substances that are foreign to the organism. Among drugs which are misused to a great extent, tablets for headache, hypnotics, and aperients are much too predominant. In a small country like Denmark, the adviser on pharmacological matters of the Public Health Authorities is able to give us the following figures: consumption of drugs for headache 150 tons; aperients 15 tons, hypnotics 9 tons – annually.

Nicotine, too, is a ruinous stimulant, a still stronger poison than spirits; it causes sclerosis of the heart and the cardiac musculature to become undernourished. The heart becomes a flaccid bag instead of a firm muscle. Many busy men who die about the age of fifty years die of heart failure caused by chronic nicotine poisoning. Here, too, I have experienced that patients on a pure, raw fruit and vegetable diet gradually lose their taste for tobacco completely.

The ground, too, is wrongly cultivated when it is fertilised too much and too uniformly with chemical manure. We may run the risk that the ground becomes just as diseased as man – over-acidified, over-nourished, and that it yields sick plants which are not fit for human food.

Raw food is termed *live food* by me, in contrast with such food as has been treated by heating, which I consider *dead food*. Care should be taken that the food does not include substances which counteract the chemistry of the organism, so that the waste products are not retained too long and putrefy in the large intestine.

The best food is therefore completely natural food which has not been subjected to denaturation of any kind.

To this must be added that live food is much easier to digest; it helps in the digestion itself, just as the living baby co-operates in its delivery. Raw vegetables have been digested in the stomach and the intestines in an hour; boiled vegetables require almost three hours and leave more waste products, also offensive stools, impure blood, and poisoned and gradually impaired organs, whereas the raw food – live food – the sunlight nourishment, dissolves and excretes these poisons.

Raw food is easy to digest; it spares and strengthens the organism in every respect, because of its content of life, bases, and vitamins in their natural, living combination and relationship to one another.

Everybody who can think, must be able to understand that our present nutrition is highly destructive – and is the most common and most serious cause of physical and mental diseases and constitutional degeneration. We must seek more wholesome nourishment and more wholesome habits of life if we are to live better now and in the future. We cannot afford to compromise when life and health are concerned. We must follow the only right way – the one hundred percent raw fruit and vegetable diet.

Let us consider for a moment how it influences our many different diseases. In the individual case it will always, on the one hand, depend on how good a constitution the patient has and how old he is; and, on the other hand, how poisoned, weakened and broken his constitution has gradually become because of preceding wrong nutrition and wrong habits.

But it may be said, largely, that if, in spite hereof, the organism is fairly fit for work and able to utilise the exclusively raw diet, the latter will exert a curative effect on almost all our diseases, both those we have acquired during our span of life and those determined by hereditary predispositions.

Even the unborn baby may be injured in various ways. The impaired germ may determine both physical and psychic diseases. The baby may be injured by the wrong nutrition of the mother, because it is nourished through the impure blood of the mother. This may pave the way for disease so that the baby is born ill.

After its birth, the condition is aggravated, mostly because the mother's milk is not as good, both qualitatively and quantitatively.

Children all over the civilised world are born weaklings to a mild or severer degree, and who can estimate the future consequence thereof? Therefore, the sooner we go in for an exclusively raw diet, the sooner and better it will exert its effect.

Children are assisted by nature, older individuals are rather opposed by nature. When a mother goes in for pure raw food, her milk secretion is immediately increased, the child thrives in all respects, the vitality is increased, and the mother can soon begin to give even young babies an addition of finely chopped fruit and vegetables; never, however, fruit and vegetables at the same time – always separately. It borders on the incomprehensible that a change can be effected so rapidly, just by giving the child wholesome mother's milk, as much as it requires, and afterwards fruit and vegetables.

I have often experienced how a large family of brothers and sisters living exclusively on a raw vegetable diet became healthy, happy, lively and nice children in the course of a few months, so good is the effect of the exclusively raw diet in childhood, which is still assisted by nature and has not yet been ruined.

The effect does not appear quite as soon in adults, but it is indisputable that raw food exerts a good effect on adults too, even psychically; it brings out equanimity and harmony, kindness and sympathy.

But what of the *elderly, sick* or the *very sick people* who have gone in for this diet too late? How about them?

Well, they have to be *patient*, energetic and very interested, and they must be able to rest much, at any rate to begin with. The first few days may be troublesome, until they have become accustomed to this different food and habit of life.

But they will soon do better; the bowels will open regularly – two or three times daily – and this is a great encouragement to many. At the Humlegaarden, garlic has its great share in this improvement. Just one clove with every fruit meal is of effect; but it is, of course, better to eat a medium-sized garlic (from five to ten cloves) with the fruit meals.

A number of works by various investigators have been published, dealing with the bactericidal effect of garlic, which people of former times guessed.

According to investigations reported in the *Journal of the American Chemical Society*, 1944, a substance known as allicin, which exerts a great inhibitory effect on bacteria, has been found in garlic.

This substance has been compared with penicillin in a number of experiments, and it appeared that allicin exerts its effects on practically all bacteria, in contrast with penicillin, the effect of which is certainly stronger but much more limited.

The use of garlic is rendered difficult because of its peculiar odour; therefore, people in Denmark often return to the Humlegaarden to undergo a course of treatment with garlic. In the company of others who eat garlic themselves, the odour cannot be smelt at all.

Raw vegetable food and, in particular, raw potatoes, exert an excellent effect on all forms of rheumatism and rheumatic arthritis when these diseases have not progressed too far.

A good effect is also seen on the diseases related to those just mentioned and of the same causation, namely, loading with uric acid; it applies to psoriasis, hemicrania, stone-formation in the gallbladder, the renal pelvis and the urinary bladder. Almost all diseases of the skin are cured, in many cases even rapidly. Loss of hair, fat formation, and dandruff cease. All infectious diseases are cured or improved.

The garlic we eat exerts an excellent effect on putrefaction in the large intestine, and a clove of garlic in either side of the mouth, placed between the cheek and the teeth, will greatly accelerate the expurgation and cure of diseases in the upper respiratory tract, first and foremost ordinary colds, if dealt with in time.

Diseases such as catarrh of the nose, the throat and the larynx, bronchitis and tuberculosis of the lungs, inflammation of the frontal sinus or the maxillary sinus, chronic inflammation of tonsils and gums, inflammation of the middle ear, and others, are cured completely in most cases. Gastric catarrh, gastric ulcer, duodenal ulcer, catarrh of the large intestine, and haemorrhoids too.

Women who carry through the raw diet during pregnancy feel well – delivery takes place rapidly and almost without pain; the slender, healthy, strong baby co-operates. The raw food produces copious and good milk for the child during the first year if the mother continues with this diet.

When a person is on an exclusively raw diet, it will, as a rule, be easy to stop smoking and drinking. Liquor does not taste well with raw food. Smoking does not agree with garlic. On an exclusively raw diet, no stimulants of any kind will be needed any more.

When cancer occurs, the organism will be, as a rule, thoroughly destroyed. Cancer is the terminal stage. Here a one hundred percent raw fruit and vegetable diet may prove helpful, alleviate the pain, prolong the life, because it agrees well with the patient. In the most favourable cases, when the cancer is dealt with in time, it may perhaps also be checked, even for many years in some cases.

I am an example of someone living for many years after the raw diet. And the treatment with raw food should be commenced as soon as the cancer is discovered, and it is an absolutely necessary condition that it is carried through one hundred percent.

I want now to tell a little about my own case from 1942 to the present year. Up to1946, I was doing well on my exclusive raw diet – the cancer of the breast was completely quiescent, and my general health was good.

But in the spring of 1946 we got some dried fruit from Sweden (raisins, dates, prunes, and figs). I thought then that it would be all right to eat it, but it was not. These are fruits which have been treated with chemical poisons in order to preserve them and to make them look attractive. Having taken them for three or four months, I suddenly developed violent pains in the scar-like tissue in the breast, and, on closer examination, I found a small node in the right breast, in the same place as before. Once more I reverted to the fresh raw food, and the node disappeared.

The last and most dangerous thing for me was, however, the trial microscopy against which I had been dissuaded by Dr M. Hindhede. I had to let it be done because so many – doctors in particular – maintained that I had never been suffering from cancer in the first place!

It was made at the Radium Centre in Copenhagen, in January 1948. This trial microscopy was positive; there were cancer cells in the scar-like tissue in the skin of the right breast, but it was a benign form called scirrhus.

My original malignant, rapidly growing form of cancer had thus, under the influence of raw food, been converted into a benign form of cancer, which remains quiescent.

But still this interference was just on the point of stirring up the cancer so much as to frighten me seriously. For the first time I developed metastases (two small nodules) in the armpit, and about six months on the exclusively raw diet were required to make them subside again.

But it went well this time.

Since then I have been in excellent health – all through last summer I was up at sunrise, and in my garden where I have been working hard several hours daily. This was far more wholesome than sitting indoors working as a doctor!

Not only had I the patients at the Humlegaarden, but also a large private practice and correspondence out of town; this was more than I could manage.

On 1st January, 1949, I stopped practising and took up gardening again, which had always been my great interest. For this purpose I had acquired about a half hectare [about one and a quarter acres] of land near the Humlegaarden and here I learned how right it was to grow both fruit and vegetables biologically; that is, according to the laws of life.

For manure, I use only compost, seaweed, straw or hay; no chemical manure, no dung.

In conclusion, just a few words about the practical conditions and the every-day use of raw fruit and vegetables. I am glad to be able to refer to my book *Live Food*, which has just been brought out by a Dutch publishing house and which gives a detailed picture of the procedure to be followed when changing to a pure raw diet.

It would be of great consequence if the medical profession would acquire greater knowledge in this field to a higher degree than is actually the case. Doctors from Denmark and from foreign countries have visited the Humlegaarden for shorter or longer periods and have utilised their experience in their practice.

The Humlegaarden is visited by about one thousand patients annually. Here the patients, as well as the members of the staff, live entirely on raw foods and our experience is that a transition diet is quite superfluous.

The raw vegetable diet can only be varied according to the seasons, and consists of three meals daily. We get a fruit meal in the morning and in the evening, and a vegetable meal in the middle of the day. Fruit and vegetables are never mixed. If the condition of the teeth permits it, the raw food is taken whole; otherwise it must be grated and reduced to small particles *immediately* before the meal is eaten.

Once the raw food has been grated or chopped, it will not keep, because it loses its content of vitamins. The raw food should be carefully chewed, preferably so well that it passes down all by itself, and even the grated raw food should at any rate be mixed well with saliva.

We drink raw whole milk with all our meals, from half a litre to one litre daily (one litre equals one and three quarter pints approximately). Germinating corn, or dried corn, crushed or ground immediately before the meal, is taken with the fruit.

Garlic is medicine and is eaten with fruit and milk, cut into small pieces in varying quantities. All kinds of nuts provide a good supplement.

The vegetable meal consists of green leaves, roots and tubers, with an admixture of a spoonful of honey. Potatoes are eaten with the peel. Similarly, all fruit is eaten with the peel. In the cases of diseases such as gastric catarrh, gastric ulcer and the like, care should, however, be taken during the initial stages.

If the exclusively raw food with its associated sound habits of life prevails, a variety of things will improve. Diseases will gradually be obviated. Obesity, the most dangerous of all diseases, will become a rarity.

The housewife's work will be reduced to half the time – and the leisure hours thus gained will be an invaluable advantage and joy for husband, children and home. The slender build, the erect carriage, the supple gait, the fresh complexion, the white, sound teeth and the vigorous hair will dominate the picture. When the body is healthy, the result will invariably be a sound mind. Our negative thoughts will be changed into positive ones, and develop the great cultural progress which the world is waiting for. *Only then will life be worth living.*

17.

Recovery From Cancer on One Raw Meal a Day
by Wong Hon Sun

The following is from the book *How I Overcame Inoperable Cancer,* by Wong Hon Sun, M.D.[41]

At the age of 32, Wong Hon Sun found himself to be a victim of a critical form (anaplastic epidermoid carcinoma) of nose and throat cancer, large and inoperable, in 1960, and, by employing principles of natural healing on his own initiative, made an unexpected and complete recovery (as confirmed by medical check-ups), with no recurrence of any symptoms of the disease for the past 14 years.

Before he began his self-care, he had a lump at the back of his throat which began to interfere with both his speech and swallowing. He was constitutionally anaemic, had chronic nasal catarrh with intermittent nose bleeds, and was extremely emaciated and undernourished.

He had radiation treatment five times a week for two weeks. This was followed by a biopsy. After the radiation, an agonising parchedness of his mouth and throat followed by nausea caused him to eat or drink nothing but occasional sips of coconut water, after which his weight dropped to 75 lbs.

His nausea ended after a three-day water fast, after which he began drinking freshly squeezed pineapple juice, alternating with liver extract every four hours. He soon recovered his strength.

He began daily walking to induce sweating for "detoxication purposes". When he returned at noon-time, he drank large quantities of the liver extract (made by steaming the liver) and fresh pineapple juice. In order to completely eliminate the toxaemia in his system, he believed that, short of complete fasting, the cancer patient may have to restrict himself to one meal a day.

"This Single Meal Routine acted as the best natural safeguard against excessive nutrient intake, while providing the minimum quantity necessary for normal physiological function. It is also tantamount to a 24-hour fast in its therapeutic effects, can be carried on indefinitely, because it vitalises (provided that the ensuing diet is of high nutritive value), rather than weakens, as prolonged fasting does."

The body adapts itself to a reduced daily food intake by lowering the basal metabolic rate, which, within limits, is favourable to early recovery from cancer, provided vitality is maintained. The resulting conservation of energy enhances the body's intrinsic healing power for the fight against cancer.

On the Single Meal Routine, he took solid liver, about 100 grams of raw liver, 3½ oz in weight (equal to approximately 30 grams of protein), which he felt he needed for his anaemia and sub-normal blood count. Also, he was unable to digest cheese, nuts, or pulses without gastric discomfort, thus necessitating the use of liver for tissue-building protein and iron.

Then, too, the use of 100% raw foods, both animal and vegetable, provided hormones, enzymes, and other vital elements needed for regeneration. To make the raw liver palatable, he immersed it in scalding water for several minutes, which made it taste enjoyably good. He gradually reduced the scalding time to a few seconds and was able to eat it with relish. This he alternated with raw eggs of various species, but mostly hen's. One day liver and the next day some eggs.

Since he couldn't handle the leafy vegetables, tubers, or nuts, he used fresh, ripe, and uncooked fruits of a softer variety. He was able to maintain his nitrogen balance on some eggs one day and 3½ oz of liver the following day. This was rather remarkable, since when he felt unwell, he always fasted on water, so that he took much less than 100 grams of liver on the average, on the alternative liver days. The balance of the diet was made up of fresh fruits, which formed its main basis.

To ensure an adequate supply of sugar, he took a few spoonfuls of honey or molasses as a dessert. On the raw liver (or raw egg) and fruit diet, he found that he was able not only to maintain, but gradually to increase, his vitality. And one day he felt energetic enough to indulge in running exercises in the open fields (more than three months after the cessation of the radiation treatments). He ran daily to sweat out the toxins – rested in the afternoon – and then in the evenings he went on a hike. Then, working up a great thirst, he would stop at stalls and have a hot beverage of boiled juices of certain melons and herbaceous plants and leaves.

At night he took a warm bath, followed by a brisk rubdown. He gradually increased the running to one, two, and three miles, and the tumour gradually regressed, and the breathing became easier. "My diet of raw liver, eggs, and fresh fruits provided me with a good supply of B complex containing B6, vitamin C, iron, and lecithin, and I further took some honey, red palm oil, brewer's yeast, and wheat germ as nutritive supplements." It took more than six months for the inflammation on his face to subside completely and more than a year for his features to become normal. The irradiated areas eventually healed, but some permanent scars remained. "I had to depend upon eggs and fish liver for my supply of vitamin D." Fish liver also contains some calcium and phosphorus, but these two minerals occur in greater quantities in egg, which also contains vitamins A and D.

Raw vegetable therapy: With gradual digestive improvement, he was able to add raw tomatoes and cucumbers and, by dipping lettuce, celery, and cabbage in boiling water for only a few seconds, they were made palatable. He juiced hard, raw vegetables like carrots. With advancing years, he reduced his intake of liver, totally excluding other animal flesh. He accustomed himself to some cheese in addition to eggs, getting a good supply of essential amino acids. He then added plant proteins, such as soybean, in the form of easily digestible curds, adding a dressing of ground nut oil.

Also added were legumes, ground nuts, lotus seeds, and natural supplements like wheat germ and yeast. As his anaemic condition improved, he took liver once a week or two weeks and relied mainly on sugar cane, beans, spinach, and other iron-rich plant foods. Thus, he gradually learned to maintain his nitrogen equilibrium without having to take meat every day. On his almost meatless and low-starch diet, he was constantly on guard against the development of hypoproteinaemia and hypoglycaemia. On some occasions he did experience mild symptoms of these conditions, but, by repeatedly adjusting his menu, he was gradually able to assess his daily requirements of protein and sugar. He always made allowance for vital food factors as yet undiscovered, so he followed no fixed menu based on known nutrients, but constantly altered his menu.

"Raw vegetable therapy, when judiciously carried out, could be a great help to the cancer patient in his fight for survival, but for the therapy to be successful, a sound knowledge of the nutrients – particularly of essential amino acids – present in various types of food is essential." Wong was convinced of the importance of auto-psychotherapy, wherein the patient understood that the human body is self-healing and the natural tendency in illness is always towards recovery (called homeostasis), provided that the causation of the illness is removed.

Faith and determination in one's recovery are essential, and if the physician can instill in the patient the faith in the intrinsic power of the body to fight off the disease, and assure him of the chances of a final victory, the best chances of success are then possible. Add to this the inspiration and confidence which comes when the patient sees progressive improvement in his condition, the gradual abatement and regression of his cancerous growth, as well as the steady increase in strength and vigour, and success is assured.

In his recovery from cancer, all his chronic afflictions which existed prior to his developing cancer disappeared – viz colds, sore throat, sinusitis, gingivitis, hay fever, indigestion, and insomnia. His sense of smell and taste gradually returned, the tumour continued to regress slowly but surely, and within eight months he was completely cleared of nasal obstruction.

He was carefully examined at a hospital and the doctor stated, "You seem to be all right. There's no trace of the tumour." He learned to avoid the cancer recurrence, which he so greatly feared, by constant vigilance. By his 35th birthday, he was so improved in health and vigour that he was able to jog for hours without feeling unduly tired. "And all the while I had adhered to the Single Meal Routine – a diet which gave me little more than 1000 calories of energy daily. On the Single Meal Routine I have been able to maintain my body weight constant at 100 lbs – not an abnormally low weight for an Asian of average height.

"This amounts to a loss of only about 10 lbs compared to my body weight in early youth, when I was eating three or four meals a day. But, paradoxically, my reduction in weight was compensated by increased vigour, a keen appetite, and – most important of all – a gradual abatement of all my chronic ailments and complete eradication of cancer."

For the past 14 years since his biopsy, free from colds, hay fever, and catarrhal troubles and in recent years, with further improvement in health and vigour, he was able to indulge in strenuous sports like badminton, judo, and weightlifting, in addition to running. "I must add that, despite my increasing daily expenditure of energy, I haven't increased substantially the quantity of food eaten daily. Yet, during the past few years, I have been able to gain a few pounds in weight."

The mechanism of human metabolism is certainly more complex than can be simply explained in terms of calorie requirements. The treatment for cancer does not end with the cure – the cure is just the beginning of the treatment. It is appalling to think of the number of supposedly "cured" cancer patients who continue to die needlessly because they won't make any personal effort to guard against recurrence of the disease!

"My recovery from cancer is in no way extraordinary or unique. The recuperative power of the human body from illness to health can only be described as little short of amazing. The cure for cancer must ultimately lie with the patient himself, and the reward of recovering is only for those who are prepared to undergo with fortitude some degree of self-denial.

"It is one of the most remarkable attributes of the human body that it can adapt itself to changes in habits of eating and living with extreme flexibility. My Single Meal Routine, initially employed as a desperate measure to check a fatal disease, has now become to me an established habit, inasmuch as I have come to look upon the three-meal-a-day routine as something bothersome and tedious. I still adhere – though it is no longer necessary to do so with rigidity – to the raw-food diet, as I consider it a natural preventative against cancer recurrence.

"My daily solo running has lost its initial boredom and become a pleasing habit. It has helped me build up a satisfactory level of health; it has helped me, in my late forties, to maintain my blood pressure at around 120mm (systolic) and to regain and relive a youth long lost to ill health and disease. To those cancer sufferers whose prospects seem dim, I would say, 'as long as there is still breath in the body and the will to live, there is always hope ... there will always be hope'."

18.

Cancer and Diet

CureZone is an organisation dedicated to "Educating Instead of Medicating". The following is from that resource:[42]

"Mark Twain quoted Benjamin Disraeli, the Prime Minister of England, as saying: "There are three kinds of lies in the world: lies, damn lies, and statistics." That statement is even more true (and dangerous) when applied to medical studies. One example is the recent Oxford University study published in The Lancet which touts the effectiveness of today's conventional cancer treatments. It supports the use of chemotherapy and states that women who used tamoxifen for five years reduced the Breast Cancer death rate by one-third.

Very impressive, until you realise that you've just been "statistic-ed"!

As presented, The Lancet cites studies proving the efficacy of tamoxifen that effectively read something like: "The National Cancer Institute's Breast Cancer Prevention Trial reported that there was a 49 percent decrease in the incidence of breast cancer in women who took tamoxifen for five years."

That's stunning. If your doctor told you that using tamoxifen cut your chances of getting breast cancer by 49%, would there be any question in your mind on whether or not to use it?

But if you look past the statistics, the truth is that, according to the study, your chance of getting breast cancer without using tamoxifen was only 1.3%. With tamoxifen it dropped to 0.68%. That represents little over one-half of one percent difference.

Then you have to factor in the dangers of actually taking tamoxifen. Tamoxifen can cause cancer of the uterus, ovaries, and gastrointestinal tract!

A study at Johns Hopkins found that tamoxifen promotes liver cancer, and, in 1996, a division of the World Health Organisation, the International Agency for Research on Cancer, declared tamoxifen a Group 1 carcinogen for the uterus. In another abruptly curtailed NCI study, 33 women that took tamoxifen developed endometrial cancer, 17 suffered blood clots in the lungs, 130 developed deep vein thrombosis (blood clots in major blood vessels), and many experienced confusion, depression, and memory loss. Other permanent damage brought about by taking tamoxifen includes osteoporosis, retinal damage, corneal changes, optic nerve damage, and cataracts. In short, the half of a single one percent of those who received a reduction in breast cancer by using tamoxifen traded it for an increase in other cancers and life-threatening diseases.

Once you look behind the numbers, is it any wonder the "war on cancer" continues to fail so miserably? The problem is that doctors themselves believe the statistically manipulated numbers that are fed to the public. And yet, the general trend is undeniable. Things are not getting better. The incidence rate of cancer has exploded from around one in five hundred in 1900 to approximately one in two today." [CureZone.com 6/6/2005.]

Cancer is a dreaded word amongst the general population, but is becoming less and less fearsome as people find natural alternatives to the standard chemotherapy treatment. Chemotherapy has a less than 5% success rate, according to the Gerson Institute/Cancer Curing Society.

Cancer was rare thousands of years ago. Nowadays, almost every family is touched by the disease.

During the Palaeolithic period, about 12,000 years ago, people ate primarily non-starchy vegetables, fruits, nuts, roots, and occasionally lean meat, including ostrich and bison, as well as organ meats and seafood – a far cry from our modern diets.

That natural diet has been largely replaced with refined white sugar, refined white flour bread, pasteurised milk and an entire panoply of processed, tinned, heated, chemical-laden, former shadows of what were once called natural food.

Our ancestors during the Palaeolithic period didn't die from heart disease, diabetes, and cancer – all the leading causes of death today.

The fact that you *can* reverse cancer – by removing the diet responsible for it and replacing it with a natural one – is still not accepted by the medical/cancer industry. They prefer to send patients down the lucrative chemotherapy route with its dismal success rate.

However, the medical establishment has been shown that cancer can be reversed by diet alone.

Dr Gerson invited the American Medical Association down to his clinic to proudly show his records of cancer recoveries, but he never heard from them again.

If you think suppression of this information is unlikely, you should realise that treating cancer by diet is a crime in America, and doctors can have their licences to practise threatened if they embrace the very idea.

It has to be realised, too, that 80 percent of Americans today – in 2012 – are eating GMOs (genetically modified organisms), and most don't even know it. I repeat – two hundred and forty *million* Americans are eating GM foods most days and don't even know it. Such is the "invisible" spread of drug-company-created GM foods throughout America. There have been no massive newspaper headlines warning people – it has been kept superbly invisible.

Keeping such a colossal impact on the general public's health quiet, and without them knowing, is a sensational piece of suppression. But it is alive and well today in America. And doubtless it will be rampant in the U.K. and other European countries before long, judging by the colossal juggernaut moving around the world that is GM foods.

If such an outrageous situation can exist – that most Americans are eating GMOs, without their even knowing it – then it should be no stretch of the imagination to consider a natural approach to healing cancer can be similarly kept from the public, by the clever use of misinformation and attempts to ridicule dietary treatments.

The cost of chemotherapy for each patient is estimated at about $100,000 in the U.S. – about £60,000 in the U.K. – maybe much, much more. With millions of people developing the condition in both countries, it is no surprise that the drug industry sees chemotherapy as the goose that lays the golden egg.

Dr Max Gerson, mentioned earlier, estimated that chemotherapy is only about 5% successful. In other words, 95 out of 100 patients receiving the treatment do not achieve a cure.

And it shouldn't be any surprise either.

Chemotherapy is famous for seriously weakening the immune system. Whereas, to recover from such a serious illness, your immune system has to be at its strongest! And certainly the only way to restore health to a human being is to feed him correctly, not pump into his body poisonous chemicals.

That correct diet can cure cancer has been known for decades, but anything that goes against orthodox chemotherapy and radiation treatments are quickly discredited and dismissed as quackery by vested interests.

But to the thousands of people who have recovered their health by changing their diets, it is a shameful indictment of medical science that they are still promoting, to this day, such ineffective treatments whilst, at the same time, fighting off claims that it is the diet of the human that is the cause of the cancer.

And, going back to what has been said elsewhere, to cure a disease you have to first find the cause and then remove it. That is not what current medical treatment does.

Japan has a low incidence of cancer. But if a Japanese emigrant to the United States adopts the American way of eating, it is not long before he falls into line with Americans and soon becomes as susceptible to cancer as Americans. However, those Japanese who emigrate to America and keep to their own, more natural Japanese diets, do *not* succumb readily to the condition!

You don't have to go far to find the cause of cancer. Our appalling diets are even recognised by the U.K. government when they themselves advise us to eat 5 fruit or vegetables a day to "prevent" cancer. Another way of reading that is that the *lack* of fruits and vegetables *causes* cancer.

Whilst medicine largely denies that cancer can be caused by poor diet, it is indeed strange that the U.K. government encourages everyone to eat 5 pieces of fruit or vegetables a day, to prevent cancer!

That is *exactly* the same as saying if you regularly consume fruits and vegetables, you will not get cancer in the first place. Yet they insist diet has nothing to do with cancer.

How much of a stretch is it, therefore, that by taking in large amounts of raw fruits and other vegetables – which the Gerson therapy advises – your body will restore its health and fend off the cancer; indeed, cure the body?

Whilst that therapy has a good success rate – far superior than any chemotherapy – not everyone will be cured. Those patients who have been damaged by large amounts of chemotherapy sometimes fail to recover on the Gerson, because the damage caused by the chemo has been so intensive.

Indeed, Charlotte Gerson, Dr Max Gerson's daughter, tries to avoid taking on patients who have been damaged by chemotherapy because, if they fail on the therapy due to the chemotherapy damage, it gives opponents of the therapy more ammunition with which to attack the therapy.

The Gerson therapy consists of 13 glasses of freshly squeezed raw, organic vegetable/fruit juices a day, along with soup and raw salads. The diet is not all raw, and that makes the diet that much easier to adhere to.

Beata Bishop, a former BBC writer, turned to the Gerson when declared terminally ill. She recovered fully to write a book on her experiences, called *A Time to Heal.* She travels around Europe lecturing on the Gerson therapy to this day.

Another lady who beat cancer, and who stated that she was making her own funeral dress when she heard of the Gerson, followed the diet and is still alive and well today, more than 30 years later. She is Jacqui Davidson, and she wrote her story in the book *Cancer Winner*.

Whilst scientists, confronted with dietary solutions to cancer, always discredit these approaches by saying the usual, "It's not scientific" or "It's only anecdotal", or saying that the person who recovered to write a book on it is not "qualified" to state 100% that they really had cancer in the first place, that is not the case with Dr Lorraine Day of California.

Dr Day couldn't be better qualified as a medical doctor.

Dr Day is an internationally acclaimed orthopaedic trauma surgeon and best-selling author who was for 15 years on the faculty of the University of California; San Francisco School of Medicine as Associate Professor; and Vice-Chairman of the Department of Orthopaedics. She was also Chief of Orthopaedic Surgery at San Francisco General Hospital and is recognised worldwide as an AIDS expert.

She has been invited to lecture extensively throughout the United States and the world and has appeared on numerous radio and television shows, including 60 Minutes, Nightline, CNN Crossfire, Oprah Winfrey, Larry King Live, The 700 Club, John Ankerberg Show, USA Radio Network, Art Bell Radio Show, Three Angels Broadcasting Network, and Trinity Broadcasting Network.

Dr Day developed breast cancer, and by using the techniques of the Gerson therapy, cured herself completely. No-one could say she was not qualified in medicine to comment. She regularly gives talks on curing cancer with diet and doubtless is the bane of the U.S. medical authorities, who still deny diet plays any part in cancer. She is often attacked by vested-interest parties upholding the false claims that chemotherapy actually *cures*! More about the Gerson therapy in a later chapter.

However, those attackers of this harmless therapy – it is, after all, just an improvement in your diet! – should be ashamed of themselves in the knowledge that they are denying cancer sufferers – men, women, and children – a real chance of recovery.

19.

Frank's Raw Diet Success

The cover photographs show how a mere 42 days on a strictly raw-food diet can transform the appearance – and, indeed, the health – of someone. The photograph is of Frank Ferrante.

Frank is living proof of the healing power of raw foods. A former drug addict and alcoholic, Frank was living with Hepatitis C, obesity, pre-diabetes, and depression.

Frank is not only, today, 110 lbs lighter, but Hepatitis-free and a vibrant image of what glowing health and happiness should look like.

Raw food can effectively regenerate your entire system, and losing weight is one of the obvious attractions of eating this way. There is no effort required, other than the simple eating of foods as nature intended, to lose your overweight. The normalising of your physiology, the melting away of unwanted pounds, is the reward for adhering to such a method of eating. The healing of annoying health disorders also comes with the territory, as has been explained throughout this book.

The old Frank Ferrante was a boisterous 54-year-old Sicilian from Brooklyn, New York, living in San Francisco. Whilst Frank loved the good life – women, good food, and a fun time – he is also a former drug and alcohol addict, living with obesity and Hepatitis C.

Long estranged from his only daughter, Frank suffered from depression, and had been single for many years. Frank was taking an assortment of prescription drugs and was constantly fatigued.

His instincts told him life surely can get much better than this, and he hoped for some miracle to pull him out of the despair.

His love of life was further diminished by his health problems, his self-loathing, and his disconnection from his family.

Frank began to visit Cafe Gratitude – a raw, vegan, and organic local cafe in San Francisco – where he found a retreat from his suffering and soon established a fast friendship with the compassionate staff. One day he was asked the question of the day by Ryland, one of his servers, "What is one thing you want to do before you die?" Frank replied: "I want to fall in love one more time, but no-one will love me looking the way I do."

Drawn to the prospect of helping the Sicilian, Ryland and two other young men from the cafe, his brother Cary, and best friend Conor, decide to personally take on Frank's healing process as their personal quest, establishing a 42-day contract with the goal of his eventual mental, physical, and spiritual renewal. All Frank had to do was put his life into the hands of the three young men and trust them to guide his total transformation, the entirety of which was captured on film, its title being *May I be Frank*.

The documentary explains how Frank begins a healing plan composed of eating a completely raw, vegan diet, doing daily positive affirmations and spiritual practices, and receiving unconditional support and love, including from himself – a difficult task, Frank admits.

These three twenty-something young men encouraged Frank's complete transformation, helping him reinvent his health, his weight, his relationships, his view of himself and the world, and his ability to love again.

Of course, it should be no surprise to anyone that Frank's health, in all areas, should dramatically improve by eating in this manner – naturally. Most overweight folk know in their hearts that, if they ate only fruit and vegetables, they would lose their weight. The difficulty is removing themselves from the long-standing habit of eating food which they consider "comfort food". And we can all be guilty of that.

But if you have other conditions, such as Frank had, then the extra incentive is there and that can make all the difference between success and failure. The combination of problems he had were resoundingly dealt with by the mere changing of his dietary from one that was unnatural to one that fully complied with the Laws of Nature.

If you watch Frank's story on film, it will empower you and undoubtedly help you understand yourself better, appreciate others, and recognise the natural beauty and instinctive healing that is within all of us. Information on the film can be had at the website www.mayibefrankmovie.com. Cafe Gratitude is located at 639 N. Larchmont Blvd., Los Angeles, CA 90004, U.S.A.[43]

20.

Man's Greatest Treasure

In his wonderful lessons in *Orthopathy* in the early part of the 20th century, Dr George Clements wrote the following, which is as true today as it ever was:[44]

"We know that the conditions supplied to man, determine the results obtained. The next step is to teach man how to supply such conditions, that his days in the flesh may be long, and filled with health and happiness.

The first great difficulty to face us, is the fact that few men are interested in the subject of health until they have lost it; and fewer still are interested in the subject of supplying such conditions, by their mode of living, as will bring them health and long life.

Most people pass blithely through their teens, with never a thought of sickness and old age. How remote 50 seems when we are 20. We feel that our vigour and power will never weaken; yet at 35 or 40 the fact of fleeting years comes painfully to the attention of many, and they then begin for the first time to realise, with a heavy heart, that they are growing old.

Let those who observe the first red streaks in the sunset of life take heed, "There is but one human machine given to our care. It can be made to run smoothly for many years, if we learn in time how to handle it. But after it is worn out – ah, then, too late! All the health information in the world will do us no good."

How many young people give thought to these things? Who pays attention to them until something serious occurs to arouse us from our peaceful lethargy? Then we abruptly face the startling fact that some terrible disorder has developed in our body.

Health is our greatest Treasure. Surround the sick man with the splendour of Croesus; let his seat be a throne of silver and his crutch a sceptre of gold; give him the precious jewels dug from the hills of the earth. Upon all these he will gaze with vain attempt, and would think himself lucky indeed, could he have, even under the smoky rafters of a thatched roof, the health of the meanest of his subjects.

Health is the natural state of man. It is far easier to be healthy than to be sickly. In spite of this fact, by harmful habits man dissipates and squanders his estate of health, as a thoughtless spendthrift wastes an inherited state of wealth. Then by the use of medicines, drugs, vaccines, serums, knives, x-rays, radium, all agencies of destruction, he hopes to recover the priceless treasure he has carelessly lost.

Millions of sufferers are searching for health. They are dragging their weary bodies from doctor to doctor, are going hither and thither trying this and that, and spending mints of money, in a frantic effort to find health.

Multitudes of the world's most brilliant doctors, still in their early years, are invalids, some dropping dead, going down to early graves. Why? Because they know nothing of the Law of Life.

For centuries, the sick have looked to medical doctors for relief. Under their care and direction, these unfortunate beings have been bled, drugged, poisoned, cut, carved, marred, scarred, and hurried on to a premature grave.

Heartbroken and penniless, bodies racked with pain, money all spent on seeking relief, by their own hand many patients have released themselves from the miseries which they could no longer endure. Disappointment and discouragement, even to a point where suicide was welcomed with open arms – this has been the terrible fate of many, who for centuries have asked the medical profession for bread, and in return have received a stone.

We all know of people who look younger than their true age; who move and show considerable athleticism which belies their real years. We know of people who, in middle age, perform feats of endurance that would leave youngsters gasping for breath.

These people seem endowed with perpetual youth. But they are not. They are ordinary people who, perhaps as a result of a fortunate legacy from good-living forefathers, or have themselves complied, unwittingly, with Nature's secrets of right living – proving that Nature is just as quick to respond favourably to those who obey her laws, as she is to exact the terrible penalty from those who do not. If we observe and obey these laws, the rewards are almost limitless; but if we disregard them, the penalty is most terrible.

By careless living, bodily disorders insidiously develop, while we allow the time to pass in which they tighten their tenacious grip upon our precious lives. Then we frantically struggle to recover, by artificial means, the vast treasure we have lost, and which no man can give back. It is gone, and too quickly comes the depressing day when the doctor frankly says that you must expect to die.

What is a year of life worth? What would you give to lengthen your life 5 or 10 years? Do you know the body is so wonderfully constructed and operated, that if we live anywhere near right, in the afternoon of our days the required amount of vital force is forthcoming to carry us on well into the late years? But no definite sign is perceived by the untrained eye that life's forces are slowly ebbing; and he who knows not the demands of Nature, may expect the grim hand of death at any time.

Nature's court room is always filled with the guilty, but cases are dispatched with amazing rapidity; for no argument is tolerated, no excuse accepted. The criminals are sentenced in droves, every second of time, and they are punished according to their works. For Nature is an inexorable Judge, condoning no faults, showing no favours.

Observe the culprits as they pass in review before the bar of this unrelenting Magistrate – thin, weak, pale, stiff, anaemic, rheumatic, neuralgic, and sad-appearing, sallow-faced wrecks, most of them. The sentences passed on some seem harsh, considering the trivial offences committed.

To one, the sentence is one week in bed. To another, three months in hospital. To another, two years on fresh fruit. Another, ten years of torture. Another, a cripple for life. To another, a forfeiture of 15 years of life. Now and then some poor wretch comes before the bar, and the Magistrate slowly draws on the black cap and solemnly pronounces the terrible sentence of death!

Recall how often we hear of people, apparently hale and hearty, who suddenly die without a moment's notice. But Nature does not, in that traitorous manner, demand the supreme sacrifice of healthy people. Even the deadly rattlesnake warns us before it strikes. Surely the Maker is not more treacherous than the despised reptile. He does not suddenly strike down, with the cruel hand of death, those of His children who observe and obey His laws. Nature warns us for years of our transgressions, before the death penalty is demanded; but in our ignorance we know it not.

Our trivial violations daily of Nature's law furnish striking similitude to the fairy falling snowflakes on the tops of the Alps. Those small specks of whiteness, singly so insignificant, frequently pile up, with quiet and imperceptible rapidity, to a height of 60 feet in one short year. This accumulated mass of snow, lying on steep declivities, forms the terrible avalanche that dashes down into the valley below, often overwhelming whole villages and destroying multitudes of lives, almost in the twinkling of an eye.

Thus, the incessant violations of Natural Law, so slight each day, accumulate in the body of the violator, all unnoticed, perchance, and then, as with the avalanche, suddenly strike him down with death, causing stupid and superstitious minds to wonder why the Creator plays such awful pranks on men.

But, as the destructive avalanche is simply the summation of many snowflakes, so the sudden snuffing out of life, almost without warning, is merely the climax of a cause of long and continued deviation from the great highway of health.

Countless thousands, who might have lived to enjoy a happy, ripe old age, fill early graves, all because of their ignorance of Nature's laws, or refusal to obey them. Approximately a million people die annually in America from doctoring for disorders which they should not have had. Legions, still under 40, die of old-age complaints that could have been prevented, did they but know how.

The conditions that we supply determine the results that follow. Our rate of dying is not a fixed matter set by so-called Providence. It is determined by our manner of living. We live long or die early as we conduct ourselves.

It is a fact, now well known, that we can increase or diminish the length of our lifespan, depending upon the way we live. Those who live long, obey more nearly Nature's demands. By learning and meeting these demands, multitudes of people have been, and are being, restored to health, and adding years to their lives, by following the examples of societies who have eaten naturally and obeyed the simple rules of common sense."

21.

Disease – It's Cause and Cure

Oliver Wendell Holmes was one of the leading physicians of America. For 37 years he was Professor of Anatomy at Harvard University. What he knew and said about medicine is worthy of consideration; therefore I quote him:

"The disgrace of medicine has been that colossal system of self-deception, in obedience to which mines have been emptied of their cankering minerals, the vegetable kingdom robbed of all its noxious growth, the entrails of animals taxed for their impurities, the poison bags of reptiles drained of their venom, and all the inconceivable abominations thus obtained, thrust down the throats of trusting human beings."[45]

He declared that medicine is a disgrace; that it is a colossal system of self-deception. At this hour the horrible substances prescribed are the great remedies of modern medicine. When this information (of natural curing) reaches every home, it hopefully means the end of this disgraceful system of self-deception, poison, and death.

The medical world has fought disease for centuries. It is searching for cures for every known disorder from colds to cancer. Today's leading doctors would truthfully admit that they have, in truth, no real cures for the overwhelming majority of diseases.

Dr Richard C. Cabot, of Boston, was recognised as one of the foremost medical doctors in American health culture. He was quoted as saying: "Most illnesses are self-limiting, in that they will cure themselves. One lists about 215 diseases known to medicine and, of these, there are about only 8 or 9 which we can cure."

Commenting upon this dismal failure of modern medicine (and it is true in the year 2012 as it ever was!), Dr W. E. Reynolds said: "The doctor does not specially list the '8 or 9' diseases that can be cured by medicine, but is that not a dismal failure on the part of medicine? Is the term 'medical science' not a joke?"

There is no disease, *per se*, said Hilden. Disease is a process of abnormal physiology. Health is a process of normal physiology. Health is the normal reaction of the body to a favourable environment. Disease is the normal reaction of the body to an unfavourable environment.

Disease is the natural, orderly function by which our vital force, under the Law of Life, strives to save the body by struggling to remove the dangerous internal obstructions, existing in the form of filth and toxins, that are depressing and hindering healthy action, or normal physiology.

Knowing the cause of disease, the remedy is obvious – remove the unfavourable environment within your body. That is what Orthopaths (Nature Cure practitioners) do, and the sick get well.

All disease is produced within the cycle of the natural workings of the body. It must be reduced in the same cycle, and by the same forces that produced it, but under a *change of conditions*.

Human ailments are removed by building health, not by the doctoring of so-called disease. Health is built by scientific biological living methods, not by using drugs, medicines, and vaccines, all of which poison and pollute the blood.

Healing is a physiological process, inherent in the body economy. No substitute can perform the work. The only worthwhile treatment is that which removes all circulatory obstructions and purifies the blood.

When the ailing body is treated in a natural manner – restoring the diet to one that is more natural for the body – its recovery is often so rapid as to amaze those unaccustomed to the body's wonderful reparative machinery.

All living organisms are self-cleansing. Our bodies strive to throw out toxins and other obstructions not natural to the system. The body unquestionably has an intelligence of its own. You only have to watch a cut on your finger heal to recognise that there is some intelligence within our bodies that strives to repair damage.

The nutritional status of your body will determine the extent of such repair. The more natural your food, the more powerful the healing reflex. The poorer the status of your nutrition, the slower the process of repair.

If you have a cut on your finger and a nurse puts iodine on it and covers it with a sticking plaster, the cut will heal. But it is not the iodine, it is not the nurse, and it is not the sticking plaster that have achieved the healing. It is the body's own in-built healing mechanism at work.

That same healing ability will work on more serious conditions, *if* the body is fed the correct nutrition to keep it in good working order. The earlier chapter on psoriasis gives a fine example of healing a life-long condition, merely by complying with natural laws of feeding your system.

22.

Has Medical Science *Really* Progressed?

The research within these pages showing you how recoveries occur when you include raw in your diet, or, better still, move on to a completely raw diet, is compelling.

Whilst science has made great progress in mobile phone technology, space travel, and other more down-to-earth areas such as computers, *medical* science, in truth, has made little progress over the last 100 years.

James Lind, a Scottish physician, who was surgeon on HMS *Salisbury* in the Channel Fleet in 1747, was the first person to discover the remarkable properties of raw citrus fruits on seamen who developed paralysis and other symptoms of scurvy on long trips at sea. It was his discovery that prompted the reference to British sailors as "Limeys".

The original cure, however, was not accepted for several decades – such was the resistance by physicians to allow something other than their potions to replace any doctor. Many sailors who developed scurvy died because these doctors simply did not know the connection between food and health – and the simple answer that was within their grasp, had they known.

An astonishing story of the sailors of the *Kronz Prinz Willem* is related in detail further on in this book. It was a German cruiser that sailed the high seas, committing piracy, stealing from ships they encountered – white flour, meat, tinned foods, etc – then sinking them. At sea for 9 months without touching land, but living off the foods looted from other ships, they developed scurvy. Doctors at the American port where they landed could not help at all. It took a newspaper journalist, knowledgeable on natural methods of curing, who managed to persuade the physicians to serve raw fruits and vegetables to the men, many of whom were prostrate. As every medical approach had failed, the doctors felt there was nothing to lose giving these very ill men, many close to death, fruits and vegetables. In a matter of weeks, the men were up and about, free from all the symptoms that almost killed them.

We may think that medical science is progressing a storm, with DNA discoveries and gene and stem cell therapy being touted regularly in the press as the answer to finding cures for this or that illness.

However, it is always the case that these are simply predictions – that the cure will become available in 5 or 10 years' time. The cure never actually comes, but the constant drumming into the general population's minds, by way of sensational headlines in newspapers or TV documentaries, impresses the ordinary person who assumes medical science offers the only hope of curing our many ills.

It was Dr Herbert Shelton, a world-famous physiologist who used fasting and diet in his San Antonio, Texas, clinic, with astonishing success, who recognised that the constant promise of medical science making advances to find cures simply did not match reality.

Dr Shelton observed:

"It is estimated that most of the drugs in use today were unknown 25 years ago. All of them, however brief their popularity, leave an aftermath of trouble in their wake. In spite of this failure to find drugs that cure chronic illnesses such as leukaemia, mental illness, psoriasis, eczema, cancer, and a host of other conditions, the search goes on night and day throughout the world for the magic bullet to cure this or that illness.

Hardly a day goes by without a newspaper somewhere in the world announcing a new wonder drug to cure cancer or heart disease, but still they search for a cure.

The rise and fall of new drugs follows a common enough pattern. Firstly, there is the discovery of the drug, followed by sensational announcements of its claims in the press and television.

Secondly, there follows the marketing and employment of the new drug with overly-optimistic forecasts of the cures the new drug is about to perform.

Thirdly, there follows a period of comparative silence, during which the drug is widely used in a wide variety of symptom complexes.

Fourthly, there follows notification of the side effects of this drug, together with the usual warning about these 'adverse reactions'.

Finally, the drug falls into disuse, as another new discovery takes its place, to follow the same course of promise, hope, expectancy and inevitable failure."

23.

The Dark Side of Medicine

There is a dark side to medicine. Scratch away at the apparently respectable surface of medical research and you will find considerable fraud, bribery, and corruption, and how drug profits are given priority over actually finding any cure for any disease.

As mentioned in chapter 1, Dr James Howenstine, M.D., states that the pharmaceutical industry has gained almost total control over the curricula taught in medical schools. Even articles published in medical journals are influenced by the drug industry.[46]

The U.K.'s NHS buys the drugs that hospitals and doctors' practices prescribe from the pharmaceutical industry. The British newspaper *The Guardian* stated that soaring drugs bills will bankrupt the NHS (*Guardian*, 29 Aug 2009). What better time than now to ditch most drugs – which almost never cure – and apply dietary approaches instead?

But certainly, the pharmaceutical industry would be far from happy if we were to cure ourselves, which would decimate their colossal drug profits. These profits are increasing year on year as we become more and more ill as a consequence of our worsening diets.

So what is happening in medical research? Why *are* real cures not being discovered?

There have been thousands of books on Nature Cure – for that is what treating disease with natural diet has been referred to over the last two centuries. And whilst the contents of many of them still hold good to this day, the readers of such books have mostly been those who were already converted.

So why, therefore, if changing to a natural raw diet cures disease, don't we all know about it?

Fortunately, it is finally becoming better known. The Food Hospital, a U.K. television programme on Channel 4, shown in 2011/2012, has uniquely become the first acknowledgement by a mere handful of mainstream medical doctors that diet can replace drugs and, indeed, cure disease. But it is still not generally accepted by the medical authorities and I suspect it will be resisted for a very long time to come. Despite even Hippocrates – the father of medicine – having quoted, "Let Food be thy Medicine", two and a half thousand years ago!

And besides that, we, in the nutritional side of alternative medicine, have been saying that food can cure disease for over 100 years, but our insistence has just been dismissed, or discredited as being "anecdotal" or "not scientific". Now, finally, they are accepting it – at least by a few of them – without any credit being given to our century of work. They appear to have "hijacked" the very idea as their own, suggesting it is new or "pioneering". We have tolerated ridicule over many, many decades, only for those physicians to finally take it on board. But they still have a lot to learn. For one thing, they insist that diet cannot cure cancer, whilst the Moermann diet in Holland, and the Gerson therapy in the U.S., have shown otherwise.

Nonetheless, if The Food Hospital brings diet cures to the fore, then excellent. Although the handful of doctors working at that hospital are still a long way from getting the whole picture. They seem to insist in isolating specific substances as being responsible for any one illness, making it appear to be a "scientific" approach, when, in truth, it is the whole natural foods in their raw state that provide any cures. No doubt in another 50 years' time they might begin to catch up with us on that one! After all, individual nutrients do not appear on their own in natural food – they come alongside many others, and their synergistic effect is what brings about any cure.

But regardless of The Food Hospital, mainstream medicine still insists on drugs as the main method of treating illness.

In the U.S., you should have thought that the success of the Gerson dietary therapy would have started an entire revolution of cancer care in America. But the very opposite happened – the pharmaceutical industry would constantly discredit it at every opportunity – almost certainly to preserve their own profits. But it appears the diet proved a threat to the profits of organised medicine and its treatments and that is why the Gerson clinic had to move over the border to Mexico, where the government were more accepting of alternative methods.

In California, it is a crime to treat cancer with diet. Medical doctors can have their careers ended if they suggest to their patients that they might be better off changing their diet rather than undergoing toxic chemotherapy when they have cancer. Only those doctors who could trust their patients to remain silent might privately tell them about the prospect of getting better with a natural diet.

In Britain, any mention to your doctor of a dietary approach to illness usually results in raised eyebrows or the stock response of, "There's no evidence it works". But when there's no desire, no will, on behalf of the medical fraternity to actually look into it, then there never will be the evidence on which they seem to insist. But this resistance by doctors and the medical profession to what should be a commonsense approach – improving your diet, therefore resulting in improved health – further serves to suppress what is a logical approach to health recovery.

DRUG COMPANY BRIBES

The drug industry has a significant influence on research, medical journals, physicians, patients, and even governments.

Monsanto, an American-based global drug giant pushing GMOs (GM foods in the U.K.) around the world, have been exposed as corrupt, indulging in bribery and fraud to get their products to market.

Monsanto's use of bribery received worldwide attention when Canadian Ministers revealed that the genetically modified food giant had offered $2 million in bribes to Public Health officials in exchange for the approval of getting bovine growth hormones put in to the Canadian milk supply. This scandal was shocking because it showed that if the drug industry cannot get a questionable hormone into the public milk supply by official means, they will use illegal means to achieve their goal – and obviously increase their profits – but at what cost to public health?

MONSANTO WHISTLE-BLOWER EXPOSES FRAUD

Former managing director of Monsanto India, Tiruvadi Jagadisan, told of how the company used to fake scientific data presented to the government in order to get commercial approvals for its products in India. Jagadisan said that government agencies with which the company used to deal in the 1980s simply depended on data supplied by Monsanto when giving approvals to their herbicides. Source: *India Today*, 9 February 2010.

Jagadisan said: "I retired from the company as I felt the management of Monsanto, U.S.A., was exploiting our country. At that time, Monsanto was getting into the seed business and I had information that a 'terminator gene' was to be incorporated in the seeds being supplied by the firm. This meant that the farmer had to buy fresh seeds from Monsanto at heavy cost every time he planted the crop."

The "terminator gene" is a feature of GM foods. It means that, rather than rice in the paddy fields reproducing itself year after year, as it has done for thousands of years, Monsanto would sell the farmer rice seeds that last only one year and do not reproduce. The farmer then has to buy more from the drug giant. Monsanto have been active in buying up seed companies around the world.

CORRUPTION

Monsanto were also fined $1.5m (£800,000) for bribing an Indonesian official to hide the environmental impact of its GM cotton.[47]

A former senior manager at Monsanto directed an Indonesian consulting firm to give a $50,000 bribe to a high-level official in Indonesia's environment ministry in 2002. The manager told the company to disguise an invoice for the bribe as "consulting fees". The GM company was facing stiff opposition from activists and farmers who were campaigning against its plans to introduce genetically modified cotton in Indonesia. Monsanto said it accepted full responsibility for what it called improper activities. The chemical giant has also admitted to paying bribes to a number of other high-ranking officials between 1997 and 2002.

MORE DRUG FRAUD

Around 90,000 so-called "scientific" drug trials, published over the past 10 years in journals, have been nothing more than public relations (PR) dressed up as research.[48]

This scam – which makes a mockery of the idea that medicine is 'scientific' – came to light after drug manufacturer Wyeth had to release secret documents to lawyers representing around 14,000 women who developed breast cancer after taking Wyeth's HRT (hormone replacement therapy) drug Prempro.

The practice is widespread – and has been for years – and has infected every prestigious medical journal currently published. Marketing and PR agencies, who have found academics prepared to put their names to papers they haven't written, have created the majority of the contents of these journals.

This strikes at the very heart of medicine, which prides itself on being an evidence-based discipline. It's clear that most studies which are presented as independent and impartial are, in fact, "spin" that has been paid for by drug companies and concocted by their marketing arms.

DRUG GIANT'S INTIMIDATION

GlaxoSmithKline (GSK), the drug company, threatened to either sue or ruin the career of a medical researcher who spoke out against its diabetes drug Avandia (rosiglitazone).

The researcher, John Buse, a Professor of Medicine at the University of North Carolina, discovered the drug increased the risk of cardiovascular disease, but his announcement of the dangers sparked a revenge campaign from GSK. One intimidatory strategy was to attempt to get his research funding stopped. (Source: *British Medical Journal*, 2007; 335: 1113).

"STAGGERING" FRAUD

Gwen Olsen, a drug industry insider, was a pharmaceutical sales rep for more than a decade. Her whistle-blowing book, *Confessions of an Rx Drug Pusher*, revealed what she learnt in her time in the industry.

Talking of antidepressant drugs, she said, "The cover-ups, misrepresentation of data, false advertising, and biased clinical research associated with the (SSRI) antidepressant drugs is staggering."

It seems the drug industry is not that dissimilar to the tobacco industry. The tobacco industry would be quite happy for you to smoke its tobacco for the rest of your life until you die. The drug industry appears to have a similar approach to business with their products.

And is that so difficult to believe? Does an ice cream seller want you to stop buying ice cream? Does a butcher want you to stop eating meat? A fishmonger, fish?

CONTROL OF INFORMATION

In 2009, *The Guardian* set up a joint collaboration with the *British Medical Journal* to present "evidence-based" medical information. In year 2011, the *BMJ* was forced to admit that it receives advertising and sponsorship money from Merck and GlaxoSmithKline, which both manufacture the MMR vaccine, following several pro-vaccine articles it had published.[49]

By this means, by collaboration with newspapers, suppression of natural treatments is subtly and almost invisibly achieved.

Of course, this "evidence-based" medical information will come from the drug industry – from research that they have carried out to validate, or not, their own drugs. But if the "evidence-based" approach was so reliable, why are drugs regularly approved then silently withdrawn a few years later when problems arise? Why should problems arise, if the evidence – the "science" – is so accurate?

If the "evidence-based" approach is so reliable, so safe, so accurate, why did they release Thalidomide in the 1960s as safe, when the resulting horrific deformities in so many children is a classic example of just how wrong this industry's drug research safety record can be?

SUPPRESSION

SWAT-style armed raids have been made on innocent organic farmers in the U.S. if their products are considered to be a threat to "food safety". The most recent raid on an organic farm was in Venice, California, at a farmers' club called Rawesome Foods.

On 3rd August 2011, a multi-agency swoop was carried out on this organic food club farm, with arrests and charges for selling raw goats' milk to their members. The bail was set at a staggering $121,000, but, after outraged public citizens held a rally on the steps of the Los Angeles County Courthouse, the bail was dramatically reduced.

When the bail was paid and the owners released, they were released only on the condition that they would comply with a **gag order** that they would give up their First Amendment Rights to free speech and agree that they would not contact the Press about the case, or send emails about it, or write anything on Facebook, etc. An *astonishing* piece of suppression.

There was also a **media blackout** put on the story. Therefore, only those who may have access to natural health websites and similar sources would even know about this astonishing assault on the freedom of speech that America is supposedly so proud of.

Far from being the danger to the public that raw milk was seen as, you will read elsewhere in this book evidence to the *outstanding health benefits* that raw (unpasteurised) milk offers.

BIASED AND DECEITFUL RESEARCH

As unbelievable as it sounds, the American Food and Drug Administration (FDA) actually *expects* drug companies to research the safety of their own drugs. The drug industry takes advantage of this by selectively publishing favourable research, discarding unfavourable research, and even manipulating results. Because the drug industry also has a significant influence on medical journals, research is typically published without the data, which makes it difficult to verify the conclusions that were drawn. Some medical journal publications are even ghost-written and published under another name.

One of the most unsettling examples of this type of biased research is with the drug Vioxx, which is a non-steroidal anti-inflammatory (NSAID) that was primarily intended to treat arthritis. Despite research indicating that Vioxx wasn't any more effective than Aleve and had the added risk of cardiovascular side-effects, Merck concealed this information and pushed the drug heavily. As a result, approximately 100,000 people suffered from heart attacks prior to the drug finally being pulled off the market.[50]

24.

Are Prescribed Drugs Safe?

It is well documented that psychiatric drugs, particularly antidepressants, can cause a host of violent side-effects, including mania, psychosis, aggression, violence, and, in the case of the antidepressant Effexor, homicidal thoughts. As far back as 1991, the Citizens Commission on Human Rights International helped organise dozens of individuals and experts testifying before the FDA (American Food and Drug Administration) that people with no prior history of violence (or suicide) became homicidal and suicidal under the influence of antidepressants. It would take the FDA another 13 years to admit antidepressants could cause suicide and black box warnings were finally issued in 2004.[51]

The drugs your doctor prescribes you are not allowed on to the market without first being tested and declared safe. But just how accurate is that testing? How reliable are such tests? In light of the statement above about the mind-altering dangers of prescribed psychiatric drugs, it is clear these drugs are anything but safe.

The never-ending list of drugs initially declared safe then later withdrawn because they prove to be dangerous is increasing all the time. And it is not just the psychiatric medications that prove dangerous after initially being declared "safe".

But how can drugs be declared safe, then later withdrawn from the market after proving to be dangerous? Surely the scientific testing is faultless? Clearly it is anything but! A classic case is Thalidomide. The horrors that came out of prescribing that drug took years to unfold, but unfold they did.

Thalidomide was sold in a number of countries across the world from 1957 until 1961, when it was withdrawn from the market after being found to be a cause of birth defects in what has been called "one of the biggest medical tragedies of modern times".

But a bigger list of drugs declared safe to be taken by humans and then subsequently withdrawn as not being so is given below. Some drugs have been withdrawn from the market because of risks to patients. Usually, this has been prompted by unexpected adverse effects that were not detected during Phase III – clinical trials – and were only apparent from post-marketing surveillance data from the wider patient community.

Withdrawn Drugs[52]

Drug name	Withdrawn	Remarks
Thalidomide	1950s-1960s	Withdrawn because of risk of birth defects.
Lysergic acid diethylamide (LSD)	1950s-1960s	Marketed as a psychiatric cure-all; withdrawn after it became widely used recreationally.
Diethylstilbestrol	1970s	Withdrawn because of risk of birth defects.
Phenformin and Buformin	1978	Withdrawn because of risk of lactic acidosis.
Ticrynafen	1982	Withdrawn because of risk of liver disease.
Zimelidine	1983	Withdrawn worldwide because of risk of Guillain-Barre syndrome.
Phenacetin	1983	An ingredient in "APC" tablet; withdrawn because of risk of cancer and kidney disease.
Methaqualone	1984	Withdrawn because of risk of addiction and overdose.
Nomifensine (Merital)	1986	Withdrawn because of risk of haemolytic anaemia.
Triazolam	1991	Withdrawn in the U.K. because of risk of psychiatric adverse drug reactions. This drug continues to be available in the U.S.
Terodiline (Micturin)	1991	Prolonged QT interval.

Temafloxacin	1992	Withdrawn in the U.S. because of allergic reactions and cases of haemolytic anaemia, leading to three patient deaths.
Flosequinan (Manoplax)	1993	Withdrawn in the U.S. because of an increased risk of hospitalisation or death.
Alpidem (Ananxyl)	1996	Withdrawn because of rare but serious hepatotoxicity.
Chlormezanone (Trancopal)	1996	Withdrawn because of rare but serious cases of toxic epidermal necrolysis.
Fen-phen (popular combination of fenfluramine and phentermine)	1997	Phentermine remains on the market, dexfenfluramine and fenfluramine later withdrawn as caused heart valve disorder.
Tolrestat (Alredase)	1997	Withdrawn because of risk of severe hepatotoxicity.
Terfenadine (Seldane, Triludan)	1998	Withdrawn because of risk of cardiac arrhythmias; superseded by fexofenadine.
Mibefradil (Posicor)	1998	Withdrawn because of dangerous interactions with other drugs.
Etretinate	1990s	Risk of birth defects; narrow therapeutic index.
Tolcapone (Tasmar)	1998	Hepatotoxicity.
Temazepam (Restoril, Euhypnos, Normison, Remestan, Tenox, Norkotral)	1999	Withdrawn in Sweden and Norway because of diversion, abuse, and a relatively high rate of overdose deaths in comparison to other drugs of its group. This drug continues to be available in most of the world, including the U.S., but under strict controls.
Astemizole (Hismanal)	1999	Arrhythmias because of interactions with other drugs.
Grepafloxacin (Raxar)	1999	Prolonged QT interval.
Troglitazone (Rezulin)	2000	Withdrawn because of risk of hepatotoxicity; superseded by pioglitazone and rosiglitazone.
Alosetron (Lotronex)	2000	Withdrawn because of risk of fatal complications of constipation; reintroduced 2002 on a restricted basis.
Cisapride (Propulsid)	2000s	Withdrawn in many countries because of risk of cardiac arrhythmias.
Amineptine (Survector)	2000	Withdrawn because of hepatotoxicity, dermatological side-effects, and abuse potential.

Phenylpropanolamine (Propagest, Dexatrim)	2000	Withdrawn because of risk of stroke in women under 50 years of age when taken at high doses (75mg twice daily) for weight loss.
Trovafloxacin (Trovan)	2001	Withdrawn because of risk of liver failure.
Cerivastatin (Baycol, Lipobay)	2001	Withdrawn because of risk of rhabdomyolysis.
Rapacuronium (Raplon)	2001	Withdrawn in many countries because of risk of fatal bronchospasm.
Rofecoxib (Vioxx)	2004	Withdrawn because of risk of myocardial infarction.
Co-proxamol (Distalgesic)	2004	Withdrawn in the U.K. due to overdose dangers.
Mixed amphetamine salts (Adderall XR)	2005	Withdrawn in Canada because of risk of stroke. See Health Canada press release. The ban was later lifted because the death rate among those taking Adderall XR was determined to be no greater than those not taking Adderall.
Hydromorphone extended-release (Palladone)	2005	Withdrawn because of a high risk of accidental overdose when administered with alcohol.
Thioridazine (Melleril)	2005	Withdrawn from U.K. market because of cardiotoxicity.
Pemoline (Cylert)	2005	Withdrawn from U.S. market because of hepatotoxicity.
Natalizumab (Tysabri)	2005-2006	Voluntarily withdrawn from U.S. market because of risk of progressive multifocal leukoencephalopathy (PML). Returned to market July, 2006.
Ximelagatran (Exanta)	2006	Withdrawn because of risk of hepatotoxicity (liver damage).
Pergolide (Permax)	2007	Voluntarily withdrawn in the U.S. because of the risk of heart valve damage. Still available elsewhere.
Tegaserod (Zelnorm)	2007	Withdrawn because of imbalance of cardiovascular ischemic events, including heart attack and stroke. Was available through a restricted access programme until April 2008.

Aprotinin (Trasylol)	2007	Withdrawn because of increased risk of complications or death; permanently withdrawn in 2008, except for research use.
Inhaled insulin (Exubera)	2007	Withdrawn in the U.K. due to poor sales caused by national restrictions on prescribing, doubts over long-term safety, and too high a cost.
Lumiracoxib (Prexige)	2007-2008	Progressively withdrawn around the world because of serious side-effects, mainly liver damage.
Rimonabant (Acomplia)	2008	Withdrawn around the world because of risk of severe depression and suicide.
Efalizumab (Raptiva)	2009	Withdrawn because of increased risk of progressive multifocal leukoencephalopathy; to be completely withdrawn from market by June 2009.
Sibutramine (Reductil/ Meridia)	2010	Withdrawn in Europe, Australasia, Canada, and the U.S. because of increased cardiovascular risk.
Gemtuzumab ozogamicin (Mylotarg)	2010	Withdrawn in the U.S. due to increased risks of veno-occlusive disease and based on results of a clinical trial in which it showed no benefit in acute myeloid leukaemia (AML)
Rosiglitazone (Avandia)	2010	Withdrawn in Europe because of increased risk of heart attacks and death. This drug continues to be available in the U.S.

Ever since the horrors of Thalidomide, which resulted in between 10,000 and 20,000 deformed babies in the early 1960s, the list of drugs initially "proven" to be safe and then going on to be withdrawn because they proved dangerous is a clear indication of how medical science and research are not the gold standard of excellence that they give the impression to be.

The safety of drugs should never be assumed, because it is only after they have been marketed and prescribed to patients that any problems can arise.

If your doctor tells you any particular drug is perfectly safe, and it wouldn't be prescribed if it were not, then look at the list above, and think of Thalidomide and all the others that have caused serious damage to patients, if not death.

The same questions should be asked over vaccinations. They originate from the same industry and if that industry gets it so wrong with drugs, then they can clearly make serious misjudgements over vaccines as well. Vaccine damage over the years has been well documented and many payments of compensation have been made. Nowadays, in America at least, the vaccine industry has somehow managed to get immunity from litigation if its vaccines damage, or even kill, children or adults.

You have to wonder what kind of influence that industry can have to get such questionable but powerful legislation put in place!

To receive such immunity from prosecution is astonishing. It is not unlike a car manufacturer selling cars, some with faulty brakes and some that are perfect, and their receiving immunity from prosecution if one of the faulty-brake cars crashes on the motorway at high speed, killing an entire family.

It is hoped that, by the time you reach the end of this book, you will have sufficient information with regard to illnesses to mean that you should only ever need to visit your doctor in dire emergencies in the future.

VULTURES KILLED BY DRUGS

It is not just medications which are declared "safe" for humans that we have to worry about. In the 1990s to the 2000s, the population of vultures in India started to reduce rapidly. From millions of the birds, which used to populate every city, they were hardly seen anywhere, with the reduction in population estimated at a staggering 99 percent.

Vultures are an important part of the eco cycle of India because, as cows are considered holy, when they die, rather than cremate them, the farmers leave them out in the open field so that scavenging vultures can consume the dead cattle.

After considerable scientific investigation, it turned out that a common veterinary pharmaceutical drug, Diclofenac, was responsible for poisoning the vultures.

It turned out that the drug, a non-steroidal anti-inflammatory drug (NSAID) given to working animals to temporarily reduce joint pain and so keep them working for longer, was responsible for the birds' deaths.

Now, this drug, as with all drugs, had to be tested and declared either safe or not. Clearly, Diclofenac joins a considerable horror list of drugs that are initially declared "safe", but, in fact, prove eventually to be lethal!

After the discovery of the connection, the drug was withdrawn from the market in India and Pakistan.

Once more, that is a chilling example of how a pharmaceutical drug, approved for animal use, is not tested for possible subsequent effects on wildlife.

Diclofenac is also known as Voltaren. It is also prescribed for human use as a painkiller. Now, Diclofenac – or Voltaren – is being linked to strokes.

In 2010, Danish researcher Dr Gunnar Gislason, of Gentofte University Hospital,[53] gave the results of an 8-year study, examining the data of more than 2.5 million Danes who were prescribed the non-steroidal anti-inflammatory drug (NSAID). The study found Diclofenac increased the risk of stroke by 86 percent in people not previously thought to be at risk.

ONE DRUG CAN LEAD TO ANOTHER

It could be called the slippery slope of pharmaceuticals: once you start taking one drug, you'll quickly need another. Researchers have outlined the familiar pattern by reviewing the drug-taking profile of the typical arthritis sufferer, who takes an NSAID for the inflammation, then a proton pump inhibitor to stop stomach damage the NSAID might cause – and the combination of the two harms the small intestine … and so another drug is needed.[54]

The new study is the first to recognise that the combination of the two drugs causes damage to the small intestine – and that is a far harder problem to resolve than any harm the NSAID might do to the large intestine.

The combination is typical in the arthritis sufferer, say researchers from the Farncombe Family Digestive Health Research Institute. The arthritis sufferer takes an NSAID – such as aspirin – to reduce inflammation and control joint pain. But the patient knows that NSAIDs cause stomach bleeding and ulcers – so he also takes a proton pump inhibitor to reduce stomach acid, and so lower the NSAID's risks.

But the chemical cocktail of the two drugs damages the small intestine, which suggests yet another drug be prescribed.

CROSS-OVER TOXICITY

There is another huge area of concern when it comes to taking medication. Quite often, a patient will have a number of pills to take every day for various ailments. The possible toxic cross-over effect of such cocktails has not been examined at any great length.

No-one truly knows the effect on any one person that such a combination of drugs may have. The cross-over effect, the combination of different chemicals, could well become responsible for any new symptom the patient gets, but neither the doctor nor the patient can definitively know, or even suspect, that the combination of drugs is the cause. Your family doctor can only go on the evidence that is supplied to him by the manufacturers of the drugs.

25.

Vaccinations

On a personal level, I have witnessed how "safe" vaccinations can be.

My own grandson had not a day's illness in his life, yet an hour after receiving a vaccination at the age of 18 months, he was screaming blue murder for no apparent reason, and the look on his face could only be described as one of being "petrified". He was hysterical.

I phoned the doctor and stated that it could only have been the vaccination, because he had never, ever been like this in his entire 18 months. She categorically refused to accept this and stated that it could only have been a coincidence!

This, from a doctor who was duty bound to report all vaccine and drug "side-effects" – or, to put it another way, *damage* – to the authorities!

This is from the *American Natural Life Magazine*:

"There is understandable concern among public health officials and parents alike as to what would happen without vaccines. In the case of at least one (the Pertussis vaccine), the vaccine, which is known or suspected of causing infantile encephalitis and sudden infant death syndrome, would appear to be worse than the disease. It has also been implicated in bacterial infections, including meningitis.

Many years ago, Sweden banned the Pertussis vaccine because of these dangers. For similar reasons, Japan delays the vaccine until after two years of age, whereas, in North America, it is usually administered at two months of age. Both Sweden and Japan are credited with having the lowest infant mortality rates in the world.

This fact would tend to discredit claims that the Pertussis vaccine is necessary to prevent an escalation of infant mortality in North America.

Children vaccinated with MMR can still get measles and mumps. In October/November 1990, clinical mumps developed in 54 students; 53 out of those 54 were fully vaccinated!

The Chicago Department of Health noted that of 186 Pertussis cases in Chicago in the fall of 1993, "74 percent were as up to date as possible on their immunisations". A large number of children are found to be sero-negative (which means they show no evidence of immunity in blood tests) four to five years after receiving the rubella vaccination. In another study, 80 percent of army recruits who had been immunised against rubella came down with the disease."[55]

From the American health newsletter of Dr Mercola, from 14th November 2009: "Increasing numbers of scientists and doctors are issuing harsh criticisms of the American government's plan to vaccinate virtually the entire U.S. population with a poorly tested vaccine that is not only ineffective against swine flu, but could cripple and even kill many more people than it helps. The CDC's public relations campaign has been running 'scare' ads that portray swine flu as a full-blown 'pandemic' responsible for snuffing out countless lives. But scientists and health officials throughout the world have called the government's claims unjustified and deliberately misleading."

Dr Lawrence B. Palevsky is an American board certified paediatrician who utilises an holistic approach to children's wellness and illness. Dr Palevsky received his medical degree from the NYU School of Medicine in 1987, completed a three-year paediatric residency at The Mount Sinai Hospital in NYC in 1990, and served as a paediatric fellow in the ambulatory care out-patient department at Bellevue Hospital, NYC, from 1990 to 1991.

He says: "When I went through medical school, I was taught that vaccines were completely safe and completely effective, and I had no reason to believe otherwise. All the information that I was taught was pretty standard in all the medical schools and the teachings and scientific literature throughout the country. I had no reason to disbelieve it."

However, Dr Palevsky began his investigation into vaccines in earnest from about 1989, because parents came to him with complaints and concerns that something had happened to their children after they were vaccinated.

Most paediatricians are indoctrinated to simply tell parents that anything related to a bad outcome from a vaccine is a mere coincidence. But, as Dr Mercola would observe: How come there are so many of these coincidences?

Dr Palevsky states: "On a personal note, I recently received the Visionary Award at the NVIC conference in Washington, DC. In my acceptance speech, I basically broke down in tears when I told the audience how I felt when I came to realise that, by routinely vaccinating thousands of innocent children at my clinic, I'd probably unwittingly caused damage to many of them. It was a very difficult thing for me to accept intellectually and emotionally.

"It is heart-breaking, because I see many of these kids who were developmentally normal, who were doing well, who were speaking, then whose voices and eye contacts were lost, who went into seizures, who developed asthma and allergies, and they had nowhere to go because their doctors told them that they don't know what they're talking about. These kids are real. The literature is showing that there are changes in the immune system of children who are vaccinated, especially if we vaccinate them before one year of age or even at one day of age."

VACCINATIONS AND COT DEATHS

Vaccinations have taken on a mantle of efficacy that is ill deserved, thanks mostly to slick PR by the drug industry, and they are regularly touted in the Press as being "life-saving". This effectively does its work, putting the fear of death into young mothers who put their entire trust in the hands of medical science.

From the Gerson Healing *Newsletter* of August 1997:

"We have long been acutely aware of the dangers of infant vaccinations. In the meantime, I should like to make our readers aware of a report reproduced in the British Gerson Support Group's publication of June 1996. In one publication (Vaccination), Dr Viera Scheibner states the following: "The diphtheria, pertussis (whooping cough), and tetanus (DPT) vaccine is given to babies as young as six to eight weeks old in many countries – including the U.S.A. It is implicated in many cases of cot death. Interestingly, in Japan in 1975 the vaccination age was moved to the age of two years, and cot death entirely disappeared."

This from the 29th August 2010 edition of the U.K.'s *Sunday Times*: "After years of reassuring parents about the safety of the MMR (measles, mumps, rubella) vaccine, the U.K. government has finally had to concede that it can have serious side-effects. A U.K. court has ruled that the vaccine caused severe brain damage in a boy, now aged 18, and has ordered the government to pay compensation. The ruling brings to an end a lengthy campaign by the boy's mother, who created the pressure group JABS to help other parents win compensation for their vaccine-damaged children. Her son was just 13 months old when he had the MMR vaccination. From being a healthy baby who was developing normally, he started to suffer epileptic fits and became unresponsive and is now severely disabled."[56]

26.

The Polio Vaccine Myths
"Polio was one of the clearly great vaccination success stories ..."
... or was it?

Leading U.S. vaccine rights attorney, Alan Phillips, researched the polio vaccine situation and stated: "It is important to understand that the polio vaccine was not universally accepted, at least initially. Despite this, polio declined both in European countries that refused mass vaccination as well as in those that employed it."

According to researcher-author Dr Viera Scheibner, 90% of polio cases were eliminated from statistics by health authorities' redefinition of the disease when the vaccine was introduced, while in reality the Salk vaccine was continuing to cause paralytic polio in several countries at a time when there were no epidemics being caused by the virus.

For example, cases of viral and aseptic meningitis, which have symptoms similar to polio, were routinely diagnosed and recorded as polio before the vaccine, but were distinguished and removed from polio statistics after the vaccine.

Also, the number of cases needed to declare an epidemic was raised from 20 to 35, and the requirement for inclusion in paralysis statistics was changed from symptoms that lasted for 24 hours to symptoms lasting 60 days (many polio victims' paralysis was temporary).

It is no wonder that polio decreased radically after vaccines – at least on paper. In 1985, the CDC (Center for Disease Control) in America reported that 87% of the cases of polio in the U.S. between 1973 and 1983 were caused by the vaccine, and later declared that all but a few imported cases since were caused by the vaccine – and most of the imported cases occurred in fully vaccinated individuals.

INCREASE IN POLIO AFTER IMMUNISATION

In New England, six states reported an increase in polio one year after the Salk vaccine immunisations. Incidences increase 642% in Massachusetts and doubled in Vermont. By 1959, 77.5% of Massachusetts' paralysis cases had received 3 doses of IPV (injected polio vaccine).

During the 1962 U.S. Congressional hearings, Dr Bernard Greenberg, head of the Department of Biostatistics for the University of North Carolina School of Public Health, testified that polio cases increased substantially after the introduction of mandatory vaccines. Although there was a 50% increase from 1957 to 1958 and an 80% increase from 1958 to 1959, he also testified that statistics had been manipulated by the Public Health Service to give the opposite impression.

In 1985, the CDCP – the Center for Media and Democracy – reported that, between 1973 and 1983, 87% of U.S. polio cases were vaccine-induced. They later declared that all but a few imported cases since were also vaccine-induced. Most of the imported cases occurred in fully immunised persons.

A FOOD LINK TO POLIO?

Dr Benjamin P. Sandler, M.D., of the Lee Foundation for Nutritional Research, wrote that Dr Sabin tells how polio occurred among American troops in China, Japan, and in the Philippines, in spite of the fact that there were no outbreaks of polio at the time among the native children and adults in those same areas in which the troops were located.

A report on polio in the Philippines in 1936 stated that 16 of 17 patients with the disease in Manila were Americans. In 1945 there were 246 cases of polio, with 52 deaths among American troops in the Philippines, according to reports to the Office of the Surgeon General. And, since the end of combat in the Philippines, polio has been among the leading causes of death in American troops; but checks have revealed no outbreaks of polio among the surrounding native population.

In fact, epidemics of polio have never been observed among the natives of the Philippines. Why has the disease been confined to the American troops in these countries?

Dr Sabin also witnessed an outbreak of polio in the summer of 1946 among American marines stationed in the Tientsin area of North China. Four men died, one was severely paralysed, and at least 25 others had non-paralytic attacks.

There was no outbreak of polio among the natives at the time. Dr Grice, a British physician in Tientsin for 25 years, informed Dr Sabin that, while he not infrequently saw paralytic polio in children in the foreign colony, he rarely saw the disease among the Chinese. The extraordinarily uncommon occurrence of polio among the yellow races living in North China was also reported by Zia in 1930.

Dr Sandler offered the following explanation for the occurrence of polio among American troops in China and the Philippines:

"The Americans took their dietary habits with them overseas.

All during the war, as soon as local combat conditions permitted, ice cream, candies, soft drinks, cakes, and the like, became available to American troops. Ice cream manufacturing equipment followed soon after combat equipment.

I saw American troops consume great quantities of candy bars when they lost their appetite for the monotonous K and C rations. It was felt that our men would feel at home, not get homesick, and have better morale if sweets were available.

Thus, I submit, polio occurred among the Americans and not among the natives because the natives did not consume the amount of sugar the Americans did."

I tend to agree with Dr Sandler. One of the symptoms of polio is paralysis. Read the symptoms of scurvy that were experienced by the crew of the *Kronprinz Willem* elsewhere in this book. Their poor diet ended up with many men suffering degrees of paralysis. Could not a deficient diet be the factor behind the paralysis in both polio and scurvy?

So could polio therefore have been a dietary deficiency disease, but because of the manner in which medical science conducts its thinking on most diseases (see the *Kronprinz Willem* incident in the following chapter), it searches instead for apparent "contagious" micro-organisms at the cellular level, whilst all the time missing the *real* cause of the illness – simple wrong feeding?

27.

Why Science Fails to Find Real Cures

This chapter effectively addresses the reason why medical science has failed to find a cure for at least 95% of all disease, human and animal. We shall start with the example of human TB and its animal equivalent, Bovine TB.

We have seen earlier how human TB has been cured by the simple addition of raw juices or raw food to the diet. But even though a cure for the disease was shown as far back as 1905 at the New York Post Graduate Medical Hospital, to this day, over 100 years later, that simple, inexpensive approach has still not been taken up by scientists.

TB is known to be a disease that is associated with poor living conditions, malnutrition and poverty. In 2007, there were an estimated 13.7 million chronic active cases, 9.3 million new cases, and 1.8 million deaths, mostly in developing countries.[57]

It is associated with malnutrition, notice. Perhaps if the focus was on the nutrition, and correcting it, we could rid our society of the disease completely.

This chapter will show that there can be a simple solution to the massively costly problem relating to tuberculosis in cattle – Bovine TB. The culling of the cattle involved is sad enough, but that is further compounded by the slaughter of badgers, despite no definitive proof that these little animals play any part in the disease.

It should be noted that Broxmeyer, a researcher into both human TB and Bovine TB, has found there are similarities in both human and Bovine tuberculosis.

Broxmeyer, a doctor who has treated TB in patients and studied it extensively, cites symptoms of TB which match the encephalopathy and neurological damage seen in Mad Cow Disease (BSE), Scrapie in sheep, and CJD in humans.

An explanation that can explain why scientists are thinking along the wrong lines when it comes to "infectious" Bovine TB, or, indeed, most human diseases, can be seen from the following story. It might at first seem completely irrelevant, but bear with me and all will become clear. Not only does the story serve a lesson on human illness, but also with regard to Bovine TB and other animal disease.

The *Kronprinz Willem*, a converted German cruiser, left Hoboken on 3rd August 1914. She roamed the seas for 255 days – almost 9 months – without touching land, subsisting entirely on supplies taken from British and French merchantmen before she sent them to the bottom of the sea.

During these 255 days, this "pirate ship" was kept very busy. She sank fourteen steamers and seized vast supplies of refined white flour, millions of pounds of fresh beef – enough to give every one of her crew of 500 men three pounds every day for a year, a considerable quantity of pork, hams and bacon, potatoes, huge amounts of canned vegetables, dried peas and beans, cakes made from white flour, coffee, refined sugar and condensed milk.

In January, the increasing pallor of the members of her crew was noticed by the chief surgeon; also the dilation of the pupils of their eyes and marked shortness of breath. But these symptoms were not considered significant, nor did anybody dream of connecting them in any way with the "high-grade diet" on which the men were living, it being in every way equal to that eaten daily by the "best people" in America.

In February, many of the men complained of swollen ankles and pain in the legs and arms. But they continued eating freely of the refined foods of high caloric value that they had accumulated from their raids. Little fruit was found on any of the destroyed vessels, not more than enough to last the crew a single day, so the fruit was confined to the Officers' Mess; and it should be noted that none of the officers was prostrated with the disease that followed.

In March, alarming conditions developed: symptoms of paralysis, dilated heart, atrophy of muscles, and pain on pressure over nerves, with anaemia and constipation, were marked.

Fifty of the men could not stand, and they were dropping at an average rate of two per day.

On 11th April 1915, she made a dash into James River, and anchored off Newport News, a floating hospital, with 500 sick men on board, 110 of them in bed and the rest coming down at the rate of four a day.

The Chief Surgeon on the ship, Dr E. Perrenon, M.D., had exhausted all his medical knowledge and the entire list of remedies that he had at his disposal. Once he ordered the ship into port, he issued a call for help.

Many important medical men, including the most famous physicians in New York, came in response to the call. But they found that not one of them had anything in their medical repertoire that would or could relieve the situation.

Then Alfred McCann, a representative of the *New York Globe*, and a student of Nature and health, not of medicine and disease, appeared on the scene. He knew what the matter was when he heard the story of the nine months at sea.

From his knowledge of Nature, McCann knew that when men are forced to live any considerable length of time on strictly denatured and cooked foods, as these men had been forced to do, with no occasional raw fruits or leafy vegetables to offset the bad diet, then illness was bound to result.

Armed with the knowledge he had attained during his studies, McCann suggested to the surgeon a list of simple, natural foods to feed the men.

To cut a long story short, the ship's surgeon did accept and acted on McCann's advice; not because he wanted to, but because it was his last and only hope.

And what happened? The results were amazing. Within ten days from the time the diet of natural foods had begun, 47 of the men were discharged from the hospital, and no more of the men succumbed to the disease.

Now, what has the above got to do with Bovine TB?

If you have read this book thus far, you will understand the importance of raw foods to human, and indeed animal, health.

Now, consider the crew of the *Kronprinz Willem*. When such a large group of men was admitted into the hospital, all with similar symptoms, what would be the prevailing thinking of our modern doctors?

On seeing such a group, all together, and all stricken down by the same disease, doctors would almost certainly consider that they were dealing with a "contagious" disease: an epidemic!

The prevailing thinking would be that they should be isolated and kept from others in case the disease spreads.

Of course, there was no such epidemic, no such contagion! But because of how they have been trained, any doctor coming across such a group of men, all suffering from clearly the same disease, would *assume* it to be a contagious disease.

But it was not a contagious disease at all; just a group of men all indulging in the same, wrong, unnatural diet, that was responsible for their ill health.

But because of their lack of training in the area of natural feeding and disease, the average doctor would assume that the disease was contagious and could result in epidemic.

BOVINE TB

Now, what has the story of the *Kronprinz Willem* got to do with the present-day approach to cattle stricken with Bovine TB?

These cattle could be the crew of the *Kronprinz Willem*. Just as the crew were eating unnatural food, so are today's cattle.

Cattle nowadays are customers of the processed food industry in much the same way as we are. Cattle are not always eating naturally. They do not feed entirely on luscious green grasses, as you would expect.

A quick look at cattle feed websites show that these companies are producing processed feed for cattle and sheep, much the same way that humans are eating processed corn flakes and other foods.

The "foods" being produced for cattle are supposedly "scientifically formulated" to meet all the animals' requirements. In the same way that packets of cereals intended for human consumption are apparently meeting all our nutritional requirements.

We should realise that, before these cereals even hit the shelves, they have been heated at high temperatures, destroying the enzymes. So much for meeting our nutritional requirements!

Cows, sheep, and other farm animals are not intended to eat cooked foods, but it appears that all the processed feeds on offer will have been heated at some stage.

On top of this faulty eating, they are given vaccines and pharmaceutical veterinary drugs and, I am led to believe, growth hormones. That entire approach is unnatural. None of this occurs in nature. It is, once again, a system of self-deception.

So I wish to propose in this book that scientists are again making the classic scientific mistake known as "circular reasoning". These scientists see the group of animals, all suffering from the same disease, and assume – wrongly – that the disease is contagious.

They are blaming a bacterium, when they should probably be blaming the unnatural diet and drug treatment the cows are given. But because their

142

training does not even address the natural diet link to health, they miss the true cause of the disease and instead find a bacterium to blame the disease on. A fine piece of circular reasoning!

Whilst the bacterium may indeed spread, it will only be the bacterium that spreads, *not* the disease itself. Much like the HIV virus is accepted as being responsible for AIDS. That virus itself can be found in people without AIDS, proving that, whilst a bacterium might be transmissible, it does not necessarily mean that it takes the disease with it. Indeed, there is every likelihood that AIDS itself is the result of faulty nutrition, knowing how scientists can home in on bacteria as being the cause of disease – completely missing the disease-causing influence of faulty diet.

Back to the Bovine TB. Whilst the care for the animals should be the simple step of feeding them natural foods, which would return them to health in due course, thousands of animals throughout the land are instead destroyed in an attempt to stop the "spread" of the disease, when in truth, no such spread will ever occur.

As science is so ill-informed when it comes to matters of cause of disease, this "contagious" thinking, this reasoning, is the automatic response by those authorised to oversee the health of our cattle industry.

I have seen some of the research into the cause of Bovine TB, as well as the human version. It all looks very impressive, but they still make the classic mistake of searching in the wrong area for answers.

They are looking for a very technical answer when the answer couldn't be more simple. Their focus on microscopic or cellular-level answers to illness means that they will hit brick wall after brick wall, but all the time making "discoveries" on the way, of "this" anomaly or "that" aberration in the structure or formation of certain aspects of physiological activity, all the *consequences* of the disorder, not the *cause*.

Let us consider the sailors who suffered from that scurvy. If blood samples had been taken from them, no doubt scientists could have found any number of abnormalities at microscopic level. No doubt new bacterium might have been observed. But they would not be finding the *cause*. Any bacteria present would have been the *result* of the disease.

So it is with cattle stricken with TB; if only scientists were to go back a few steps, to consider what the animals had been fed, then they could have found the real answer. But they get so bogged down in the wrong area of research that they have managed to make an entire science out of looking in wrong areas.

Let us consider an analogy. We have an international athlete, a 400m hurdler say, who might be favourite to win an Olympic gold, but who finishes last in his heat, not even reaching the final.

Subsequent investigation by his coaches into what went wrong or where his technique let him down would be avidly pursued. Every take-off would be closely examined, every clearing of every hurdle, every landing, would all be looked at and compared to previous races that he might have won. The way he held his head, the movement of the shoulders, his arm technique, the bending of his knees, all would be thoroughly inspected to find out what went wrong. But all that investigation counted for nothing when it would turn out that the athlete had taken a Valium an hour before the race to calm him down, which was the reason behind his poor performance. His coaches had been missing the *real* cause of the problem. They were looking in the wrong area. So it is with researchers into TB and other diseases.

Returning to Broxmeyer's work, Broxmeyer and other researchers assessed the antimicrobial efficacy of *Mycobacterium smegmatis* organisms carrying the lytic TM4 phage virus, introducing these virus-laden microbes into tuberculosis-infected macrophage cultures.

Is that impressive? Of course. Scientific? It appears to be. Relevant? In my opinion, no, as it misses the actual cause of Tuberculosis.

A simple change in the eating pattern of TB sufferers, whether human or animal, and the need for all this scientific research would vanish in an instant.

So, will this approach to Bovine TB and indeed other diseases discussed in this book, be taken up by scientists, and a new paradigm of health treatment followed? Of course not. It is not scientific enough! It is too simple; too low-tech. Apparently, even if something works, it will not be accepted unless it meets with completely wrong scientific criteria!

It will never be accepted, for the shake-up in their belief system would be too much to tolerate. The entire medical, pharmaceutical, and veterinary systems and their education would need to be overhauled; if it didn't collapse entirely, that is. And the subsequent loss of worldwide profits for its drugs and vaccines wouldn't bear thinking about.

And, as a timely reminder at this point in the book, and just to re-emphasise how unnatural it is to eat cooked foods, remember back to chapter 1, wherein Dr Kouchakoff showed that, when we eat cooked foods, digestive leukocytosis occurs. But this increase in the number of white blood cells (an indicator of a disease process of some kind within the body) does *not* occur on a raw-food diet.

28.

Dr Weston A. Price

In the 1930s, a Cleveland dentist named Weston A. Price (1870-1948) began a series of unique investigations. For over ten years, he travelled to isolated parts of the globe to study the health of populations untouched by Western civilization.

He wanted to discover the factors responsible for good dental health. His studies revealed that dental caries and deformed dental arches resulting in crowded, crooked teeth are the result of nutritional deficiencies, not inherited genetic defects.

The groups Price studied included sequestered villages in Switzerland, Gaelic communities in the Outer Hebrides, indigenous peoples of North and South America, Melanesian and Polynesian South Sea Islanders, African tribes, Australian Aborigines and New Zealand Maoris.

Wherever he went, Dr Price found that beautiful straight teeth, freedom from decay, good physiques, resistance to disease and fine characters were typical of native groups on their traditional raw diets, rich in essential nutrients.

These healthy races, Weston Price observed, ate mostly raw foods and only ate meat occasionally.

The isolated people Price photographed – with their fine bodies, ease of reproduction, emotional stability, and freedom from degenerative ills – are in sharp contrast to our "civilised" modern people, subsisting on the foods of modern commerce, such as white refined sugar, white flour, pasteurised milk, and convenience items filled with all manner of additives, preservatives, stabilisers, etc, in order to extend shelf-life and thereby increase profit.

The discoveries and conclusions of Dr Price are presented in his classic volume, *Nutrition and Physical Degeneration*.[58] The book contains striking photographs of handsome, healthy, primitive people and illustrates in an unforgettable way the physical degeneration that occurs when human groups abandon nourishing traditional diets in favour of modern convenience foods.

29.

Civilised vs Primitive Health

There has been a lot written about the state of human health in civilised society. Most of it is couched in optimistic terms, describing modern medical advances involving the development of new drugs, stem cell research, organ transplants, and other medical modalities.

However, in truth, results have been less spectacular and impressive than we have been led to believe, and the true picture is far from hopeful or optimistic.

All indications point to a very low standard of health for our "civilised" populations, with chronic illness of all kinds on the rise as never before. Cancer, heart disease, obesity, diabetes – all are on the rise. Medical science has made no reduction in these statistics, despite daily pronouncements of this research and that research promising a cure in ten or so years.

This drip, drip, drip of almost daily medical pronouncements serves the medical industry well, in that it slowly brainwashes the general public into believing that medical science has, or will have, all the answers to our mounting epidemic of illness. The impressive medical terminology, going over the heads of the average reader of any newspaper, serves to instil a feeling of confidence in the progress of medicine. However, that confidence is ill-founded.

In the U.S. and Europe – the most "civilised" areas of our planet – we can find examples of human deterioration manifesting themselves on a scale until now unknown in the realms of biology and medicine.

What exactly are the characteristics of the physical and mental degeneration of modern man? They are: dental decay, deformity of the dental arch, defective facial and body form, impaired reproductive efficiency, low immunity to many infectious diseases, cancers, heart disease, obesity, arthritis, early deaths, and a host of nervous or mental disorders, increasing year on year.

Add to that mix the toxic implications to our bodies of drugs prescribed to "restore health", and the list of complaints climbs and climbs.

It is claimed that we are living longer, that many of us will live to see 100. Because of improvements in hygiene, there are less deaths in infancy or at birth. When such early deaths are removed from the statistics, then we will arrive at a longer lifespan – because of simple mathematics. But if we truly are living longer, it will only be by a few years, and even then we will encounter an old age riddled with general poor health, with arthritis, angina perhaps, painful conditions, and symptoms of senility such as Alzheimer's disease – yet another degenerative condition on the increase – not to mention a growing incidence of suicide.

Mental illnesses have also rocketed in recent decades, and with the only treatment available being toxic drugs, often worsening the conditions, then the incidence of such despair will inevitably increase much further.

We now live in a world riddled with chronic health complaints of all kinds. We – and that includes doctors and scientists – can no longer visualise the nature of robust health and the conditions necessary for its presence.

To find true health, you have to visit the primitive societies who, until visited by outsiders who changed the primitives' diets by the introduction of white flour and the like, experienced health and happiness in abundance. They ate foods that were not tampered with or refined. Nutrients were not removed from their foods so that they would last longer on the supermarket shelves. The heating of their natural foods was virtually unknown and most of their dietary was consumed raw. Most of our foods in supermarkets have been, in the processing of getting there, heated.

The following reports should be a lesson in humility to our medical scientists – as well as a lesson in science itself. These reports should give a stand-out reason why we, in today's society, are so condemned to a life of misery and illness.

And it is the interference of our food with cooking which is the primary cause. Behind that, we have drugs pumped into animals which we then consume when we eat those animals; chemicals sprayed on to our foods and the soil from which our food grows; and all manner of additives that no primitive, healthy society would ever encounter.

We are the makers of our own misfortune, and the sooner we realise that, and deal with it, the better.

The following reports should alert our scientists to what life really *could* be like, if only we were to put human health first and not profit.

30.

Societies Living on Raw Food
– the Marquesa Islanders

Whilst we, in our modern cities, can only guess at how we would feel and look if we were to live pretty much exclusively on a raw fruit and vegetable diet, there are examples to which we may look to see just what would be in store for us.

It is those societies – who are isolated from so-called civilisation (or *were* isolated before being visited by outsiders) – who can show us just what life was like on such a dietary regimen.

Among the most handsome and interesting of the primitive races are the Polynesians, a strong and well-formed people living on the romantic islands of the South Seas.

Their normal characteristics are oval features, dark hair either straight or curly, a complexion of pale golden colour, height exceeding the average, pleasant dispositions, and facial features somewhat between the Caucasian and Malay in form.

Approximately 160,000 members of this race lived on an archipelago of 13 volcanic islands, known as the Marquesas, located near the Equator in the South Pacific Ocean.

The Marquesas have long been known as the most beautiful and picturesque of the South Sea Islands, and their inhabitants had the distinction of being physically the most perfect of all the Polynesians, thus being pre-eminent among many fine racial groups.

The Marquesans lived in their primitive state primarily upon tropical fruits and plants. These grew profusely in the genial climate of the area, and nearly all trees on the islands yielded fruit or other edible produce.

The stately breadfruit tree, which was indigenous to some extent in nearly all Polynesian lands, attained its greatest excellence in the islands of the Marquesas group, where it was found in fully 52 varieties and flourished in the utmost abundance.

The breadfruit itself formed the principal article of food for nearly all of the natives. Coconut and bananas were next in importance, in the order named, with the former being usually consumed in its immature state, when it was rich in fluid and of a soft jelly-like texture.

The banana was found in different sizes and types, there being nearly thirty vane types of this fruit on the islands. For vegetable roots, the people used taro, supplemented by yams and sweet potatoes.

Sugar cane was consumed in moderate amounts. (Note: This would be raw, natural sugar, and not processed sugar: Ed). The Marquesans did not till their soil, and, though some of the trees and plants were given special care, the plant foods in general were obtained in their wild state, as the bountiful nature here supplied them.

Of animal foods, the Marquesans were passionately fond of raw fish, which were rapidly devoured just as soon as they were taken from the sea. The fish were consumed in their whole state, including the head, eyes, scales, bones, gills, and internal organs.

Other animal foods used by the Marquesans were fowl and pork, though these did not figure largely in their diet. The fowl were rarely eaten, but were kept chiefly for the sake of their feathers, which were plucked out and used for decoration or ornament.

The hogs were allowed to roam at large in the fruit and coconut groves, and on special occasions – the birth of a child, a wedding or funeral, the tattooing of a person of distinction, and certain large dances and festivals – some of them would be killed and eaten at the associated feast. Among a number of the tribes, however, the pork was taboo to the women and eaten only by men of the privileged order of society.

The Marquesan diet was very largely raw. In addition to fish, the young coconuts and many of the fruits were used without cooking or other culinary preparation. Taro roots were often grated and mixed with coconut oil; sugar cane was chewed in its raw state, and sometimes the juice would be extracted and consumed.

Fresh breadfruit was usually roasted for ten to fifteen minutes on the embers of a fire, whereas various breadfruit puddings were baked for a short period on the hot stones of underground ovens. The latter method was also commonly used in the preparation of certain other foods, in particular yams and pork.

The first explorers to arrive at the Marquesas Islands called the people the healthiest and most beautiful in the world. Never before or since has a racial group been so enthusiastically extolled for its excellence of physical development.

Glowing accounts told of the natives' superb physiques, fine countenances, very attractive facial features, and vivacious, happy dispositions.

Some of the men were said to display the torsos and arms of veritable giants; the women were smaller, of delicate development and matchless perfection of form.

The Marquesan teeth were described as pearly-white, completely immune to decay, and of perfect regularity. The people were said to live to great age and were strong and vigorous in advanced years.

Travellers wrote with almost poetic delight of this paradise of song, games, swimming, dancing, mirth and laughter. Some of the early navigators were so impressed by the health and happiness of the people, that they reported the islands as the Garden of Eden!

The testimony from the past, which illustrates the Marquesan physical superiority, commences with that derived from the voyage of Alvaro de Mendana, a navigator of the Spanish Viceroy. Mendana discovered four of the Marquesas Islands in 1595, and he made landing expeditions on each of them.

His second in command, Fernandez de Quiros, was chronicler of the voyage, and three other Spaniards – Sanvitores, Figueroa and Mendoza – also left notes telling of their observations on the islands. All described the natives as finely formed and beautiful to behold, with Quiros leaving us the following description of the approach to Magdalena, the first island to be seen, and the impression made by the first natives who came to meet the ship:

"On the following day, without doubt whether that island was inhabited, the ships were steered to the south of it, and very near the coast. From a point under the peaked hill towards the east end, there came out seventy small canoes, not all the same size, made of one piece of wood, with outriggers of cane on each side, after the manner of the gunwhales of galleys, which reach to the water on which they press to prevent the canoe from capsizing, and all their paddles rowing. The least number they had in a canoe was three, the greatest ten, some swimming and others hanging on – altogether, four hundred natives almost white, and of very graceful shape, well-formed, robust, good legs and feet, hands with long fingers, good eyes, mouth and teeth, and the same with the other features. Their skin was clear, showing them to be a strong and healthy race, and indeed robust.

They all came naked, without any part covered; their faces and bodies in patterns of a blue colour, painted with fish and other patterns. Their hair was like that of women, very long and loose, some of it twisted, and they themselves gave it turns. Many of them were ruddy. They had beautiful youths who, for a people barbaric and naked, it was certainly pleasant to see, and they had much cause to praise their Creator."

On another island to be observed, Santa Christina, Quiros informs us that: "The Chief Pilot did not see anything of the women because he did not land at the time that they came; but all who saw them reported that they had beautiful legs and hands, fine eyes, fair countenances, small waists, and graceful forms, and some of them prettier than the ladies of Lima, who are famed for their beauty."

Sanvitores reported that the people of this race "remain in good health to an advanced age and it is very normal to live ninety to one hundred years". Figueroa found the Marquesan men to be "well made, and of good stature", and he observed the young boys to have "beautiful faces and the most promising animation of countenance". He noted the women to be "extremely beautiful", having "delicate hands, a good shape, and slender waists".

Mendoza stated that the Marquesans were "light-complexioned people of pleasing and regular features", with some of the men being "as large as giants, and of so great strength, that it has actually happened that one of them while standing on the ground, has laid hold of two Spaniards of good stature, seizing each of them by one foot with his hands and lifting them thus as if they were children".

Mendana left the Marquesas on 5th August of the year of their discovery, and the islands were not visited again for nearly two centuries.

In 1774, the illustrious Captain Cook rediscovered the group, with the addition of the island of Fatahuka. He found the natives to be the most beautiful he had ever seen, and he stated: "The inhabitants of these islands, collectively, are without exception the finest race of people in this sea. For good shapes and regular features, they perhaps surpass all other nations."

During the next score of years, a number of other prominent navigators stopped at the Marquesas Islands, and the northern section of the island group was first observed by an American, Captain Ingraham, in 1777.

The first missionary ship to arrive at the islands was the British vessel, *Duff*, which came in 1797 and left one missionary in the area. Captain

Wilson was commanding officer of the ship, and when three miles from shore he noted his first visitors: "They were seven beautiful young women, swimming quite naked, except for a few green leaves tied round their middle; they kept playing round the ship for three hours."

The first taken on board was described as "offering such symmetry of features, as did all her companions, that as models for the statuary and painter their equal can seldom be found".

Upon landing and observing the general population, Captain Wilson also made many insertions in his journal account that are pertinent for this study. As examples: "The women at the Marquesas, for beauty of feature, symmetry of form, and lightness of colour, far exceeded the other islands. ... Their diseases are few; I have indeed hardly observed the appearance of any. ... Not a single deformed or ill-proportioned person was seen on the island; all were strong, well-limbed and remarkably active. ... Their countenances are pleasing, open, and display much vivacity."

In 1804, the Russian explorer, Captain Krusenstern, stopped at the Marquesas Islands and visited the island of Nukuhiva. Here he made a considerable study of the inhabitants and gave these notations as to their physical well-being: "The Nukuhivers are invariably of a large stature, and well made; they are very muscular, with a long handsome neck; have a great regularity of countenance; and an air of real goodness which was not belied by their dealing with us. ... These islanders are besides remarkable for having no deformed persons among them, none of us at least saw any, and their bodies are besides free from hues and sores. ... The Nukuhivers are in the enviable possession of the most constant health, and they have hitherto been so fortunate as to escape the venereal disease; as they are free from complaint, so are they ignorant of all medicine."

During the following year, another Russian voyager, George von Langsdorff, entered the Marquesas area and carried out an extensive investigation of the archipelago. Whilst stationed near one of the islands, at the time of his arrival, he made these observations:

"A number of islanders came from the opposite shore of the harbour, which was to the northwest, and swam to the place where we were anchored, a distance of three miles. At first we could only see a shoal of black-haired heads just above the water, but in a short time we had the very extraordinary spectacle presented us of some hundred men, girls and boys, all swimming about the ship, having in their hands coconuts, breadfruit and bananas, which they had brought to sell.

The cries, the laughter of these mirthful people was indescribable, and made a very novel impression upon us. Only a few, whom Roberts pointed out as persons of distinction, were invited on board; the rest swam and played about like a group of Tritons."

On land, Langsdorff noted that the Marquesans "excel in beauty and grandeur of form, in regularity of features, all the other South Sea Islanders".

The people's expression of countenance was "generally pleasing" and "open and animated".

The women were found to be much smaller than the men, but they were said to be "extremely well proportioned", being "of form, with slender waists and great vivacity, so that they had just cause to be called handsome". They have "well-formed heads, their faces are rather full and round, rather than long, they have large sparkling eyes, clear complexions, very fine teeth, great expression and regularity of features and generally black curly hair".

Of the other sex, Langsdorff had this to say:

"The men are almost all tall, robust and well made. Few were so fat and unwieldy as the Tahitians, none so lean and meagre as the people of Easter Island. We did not see a single cripple or deformed person, but such regularity of form, that it greatly excited our astonishment.

Many of them might very well have been placed by the side of the most celebrated masterpieces of antiquity, and they would have lost nothing by comparison.

Their beards are commonly shining, black, and thin, as they are very much in the habit of plucking up the hairs by the roots. The hair is generally long, curly, strong and black; among a few it was less black.

A certain Mau-ku-u, or Mafau Tapautakava, particularly attracted our attention from his extraordinary height, the vast strength of his body, and the admirable proportion of his limbs and muscles. He was now twenty years old, and was six feet, two inches high, Paris measure, and Counsellor Telesius, who unites the eye of a connoisseur and an artist, said he never saw one so perfectly proportioned. He took the trouble to measure every part of this man with the utmost exactness, and after our return to Europe imparted his observations to Counsellor Blumenbach, of Gottingen, who has studied so assiduously the natural history of man.

This latter compared the proportions with the Apollo of Belevedere, and found that those of the masterpiece of the finest ages of Grecian art, in which was found every possible integer in the composition of manly beauty, corresponded exactly with our Mafau, an inhabitant of the island of Nukuhiva.

We were told that the chief of a neighbouring island, by the name of Upoa, with equally exact proportions as Mafau, was at least a head taller, so at least Roberts and Cabri both assured us; if they were correct, this man must be nearly seven Paris feet high."

Regarding other observations on the Marquesas Islands, Langsdorff noted that the women experienced very easy delivery in childbirth, with labour usually lasting about a half-hour.

The children were not weaned until they were able to speak or go about alone, and fruits and raw fish supplemented the milk fare in these early years.

The people were found to have an extreme facility in climbing trees and steep rocks, but it was in the sea that they displayed the most incredible celerity. They learned to swim when mere infants, and many of the adults would spend half their waking hours in the water.

A number swam about the ship for the greater part of the day, without ever appearing tired. They would even eat meals in the water, having the coconut, breadfruit and bananas tied on the end of a stick, which each would carry to sea.

Thus guiding themselves solely by the feet, they could easily shell and eat a coconut. Some of the women swam with little children on their shoulders, and others would think nothing of throwing themselves from high rocks and cliffs into the water. Some of the men ran up the main mast of the ship many times, and hurled themselves from it into the sea in a frenzy of delight and pleasure.

The Marquesans were impressive to Langsdorff, and they were equally so to the American, Commodore David Porter, who saw them in 1818. Commodore Porter visited different islands in the group, but spent most of his time in the valleys of Happa, Shoeume and Hannahow, in Nukuhiva.

Here he observed thousands of natives, and stated that "a more honest or friendly and better disposed people does not exist under the sun".

He noted that "all are in health and vigour; old and young are active and strong". Regarding the general characteristics of the people, he pointed out:

"They have been stigmatised by the name of savages; a term wrongly applied; they rank high on the scale of human beings, whether we consider them morally, or physically. We find them brave, generous, honest, benevolent, acute, ingenious, and intelligent, and the beauty, and regular proportions of their bodies correspond with the perfections of their minds. They are far above the common stature of the human race, seldom less than five feet eleven inches, but most commonly six feet two or three inches, and in every way proportioned. Their faces are remarkably handsome, with keen, piercing eyes; teeth white, and more beautiful than ivory; countenances open and expressive, which reflect every emotion in their souls; limbs which might serve as models for a statuary, and strength and activity proportioned to their appearance."

The women were described by Porter as "possessing open and intelligent countenances, fine eyes and teeth, and much acuteness and vivacity. Their limbs and hands are much more beautifully proportioned than those of any other women."

The young girls "were handsome and well formed, their skins were remarkably soft and smooth, and their complexions no darker than many brunettes in America, celebrated for their beauty".

Other American travellers to visit the Marquesas, and see the natives in their primitive state, were the naval officers, Captain Fanning and Captain Finch. The former observed natives in the northern part of the island group, and he found all the men to be "well formed and exceedingly active, either on land or in the water", with both sexes having "excellent teeth, as white and sound as one could declare possible".

Captain Finch and his party went into Happa Valley, and the chaplain, Stewart, reporting on the trip, noted that the natives were "decidedly a finer and more handsome looking people than the Society or Sandwich Islanders".

He described the women as being "exceedingly beautiful", and observed that "in figure, they are small and delicately formed, with arms and hands that would bear comparison with any in the drawing rooms of the most polished noblesse. ... Their eyes have a rich brilliancy, softened by the long glossy eyelashes that can scarce be surpassed, which with a regularity and whiteness of teeth unrivalled, add greatly to the impression of features of a more European mould than most uncivilised people I have seen."

Few writers have touched upon the Marquesas Islands with the genius of Herman Melville. This celebrated writer of the 19th century saw the Marquesas in 1844 during a four-month residence in the Typee Valley (adjoining Happa Valley) of Nukuhiva Island.

The residing natives were about two thousand in number. They were known as a war-like people who resisted the influx of civilisation, and their valley was one of the last parts of the island to become civilised.

At the time of Melville's visit, they were still living under conditions of comparative isolation, and some of them had never before seen a white man.

Melville described the Typees in eloquent and poetic terms and found them to be magnificent examples of physical perfection. One of the young girls, by name Fayaway, especially attracted his attention, and her description, which "will in some measure apply to nearly all the youthful portions of her sex in the valley", is here given in part:

"Her free pliant figure was the very perfection of female grace and beauty. Her complexion was a rich and mantling olive, and when watching the glow upon her cheeks I could almost swear that beneath the transparent medium there lurked the blushes of a faint vermillion.

The face of the girl was rounded oval, and each figure as perfectly formed as the heart or imagination could desire. Her full lips, when parted with a smile, disclosed teeth of dazzling whiteness; and when her rosy mouth opened with a burst of merriment, they looked like the milk-white seeds of the "arta", a fruit of the valley, which, when cleft in twain, shows them reposing in rows on either side, imbedded in the rich and juicy pulp. Her hair of the deepest brown parted irregularly in the middle, flowed in natural ringlets over her shoulders, and, whenever she changed to stoop, fell over and hid from view her lovely bosom. Gazing into the depths of her strange blue eyes, when she was in a contemplative mood, they seemed most placid yet unfathomable; but when illuminated by some lively emotion, they beamed upon the beholder as stars."

Melville also described the "matchless symmetry of form" of one of the men. "His unclad limbs were beautifully formed; the elegant outline of his figure, together with his beardless cheeks, might have entitled him to the distinction of the Polynesian Apollo; and indeed the oval of his countenance and the regularity of every feature reminded me of an antique bust. But the marble repose of art was supplied by a warmth and liveliness of expression only to be seen in the South Sea Islander under the most favourable development of nature. The hair of Marnoo was a rich curling brown, and twined about his temples and neck in close curling ringlets, which danced up and down continually when he was animated in conversation."

But it was not only in certain individuals that such physical excellence was found. At one of the many dancing festivals, where nearly all inhabitants of the valley were gathered, Melville noted:

"In beauty of form they surpassed anything I had ever seen. Not a single instance of natural deformity was observable in all the throng attending the revels.

Occasionally I noticed among the men the scars of wounds they had received in battle; and sometimes, though very seldom, the loss of a finger, or an eye or an arm, attributable to the same cause. With these exceptions, every individual appeared free from those blemishes which sometimes mar the effect of an otherwise perfect form.

But their physical excellence did not merely consist in an exemption from these evils; nearly every individual of their midst might have been taken for a sculptor's model."

On yet another occasion, Melville observed: "Nothing in the appearance of these islanders struck me more forcibly than the whiteness of their teeth. The novelist always compares the masticators of his heroine to ivory; but I boldly pronounce the teeth of the Typees to be far more beautiful than ivory itself. The jaws of the oldest greybeards among them were much better garnished than those of most of the youth in civilised countries; while the teeth of the young and middle-aged in their purity and whiteness, were actually dazzling to the eye."

Melville referred to the "light-hearted joyousness and continual happiness" that everywhere prevailed in the valley. This, he thought, sprung principally from "the mere buoyant sense of a healthful physical existence. And indeed in this particular the Typees had ample reason to felicitate themselves, for sickness was almost unknown.

"During the whole period of my stay I saw but one invalid among them; and on their smooth clear skins you observed no blemish or mark of disease."

Melville provided one of the last descriptions of Marquesan life as it still existed under the age-old customs of the race. There were, however, some Marquesans that remained in isolation, living upon native foods, throughout the following years and indeed up to the 20th century.

In the early 1920s a group of these were found living on one of the islands, and they were extensively photographed for the travel film, *Gow*, covering primitive life on the South Sea Islands. The splendid health, perfect physiques and great vivacity and happiness of these natives were then given vivid illustration. In more recent years the number of individuals living entirely on native foods has doubtless further decreased, and on the islands visited by Dr Price in 1934, only a few remained for observation.

With the exceptions mentioned, the general Marquesan population has followed a historical pattern similar to that of other primitive races, with most sections of the islands being subjected to the influences of civilisation even prior to and during the reign of Melville's residence. In the vicinity of Nukuhiva Bay, where there was much commerce between Europeans and natives, Melville noted that the people were addicted to civilised vices, suffered from disease, and were much inferior in physical strength and beauty to the inhabitants of Typee Valley.

Missionaries had arrived and were busily engaged in the process of saving the natives from the gods of their traditional antiquity.

European clothing was replacing, by force of missionary demands, the nudity and semi-nudity of the past.

Special foods were imported for use by the missionaries, and soon the natives were using them too. Trade ships brought in tea, salt, biscuits, syrup, sugar, flour and liquor. Opium was shipped to the islands in large amounts to please the immigrant Chinese, and its use quickly spread among the natives.

The change in Marquesas proceeded gradually throughout the years, and today it may be seen in its total culmination.

The modern Marquesan has largely ceased to depend upon the sea for food, and few of the staple plant foods known in the past are ever eaten.

The basic portion of the diet now consists of white flour products, refined sugar and other modern foods, which are obtained from trade ships in exchange for the native production of cotton, coffee, vanilla and copra.

Throughout the past century, writers and travellers have told of the Marquesas Islands and the tremendous changes, both physical and mental, affecting the native people. Just as soon as the new foods and civilised vices came into use in a respective district, then the people became ill and rapidly died.

In Happa Valley, for instance, the group of people described in such moving terms by Porter and Stewart gradually submitted later to the introduction of civilised ways. In 1888, the visiting poet, Robert Louis Stevenson, reported them to have been very nearly wiped out by smallpox, tuberculosis and other diseases. Only two survivors, a man and woman, remained to flee from the newly created solitude. [Note: You will read elsewhere in this book how tuberculosis is a product of wrong long-term feeding and that it can be corrected by the patient being provided with either a part-raw or wholly-raw diet. Ed]

So deadly were the (then thought) infectious diseases in the Marquesas that only 52,000 of the natives were still living at the time of the 1842 census; 4,000 were counted at the beginning of the 20th century, and today less than half that number – scarcely one percent of the original population – remain.

They are a sick and dying primitive group, struggling to maintain their existence and preserve their race. The French government supplied them with a hospital, four leper asylums, modern dispensaries and advanced medical services, but this seems to be of no avail in the face of innumerable diseases that strike.

Measles and certain other infectious ailments are less common than formerly, but tuberculosis remains a serious problem, and about ten percent of the natives exhibit symptoms of the disease. Few of the islanders retain a clear and smooth skin, and various forms of skin eruptions and ulcerations, in particular leprosy, are frequently seen.

Physical deformity is not uncommon, with the average stature of the people no longer reaching the lofty proportions of former days. The most striking change, however, is to be seen in the condition of the teeth, for dental decay is rampant and discoloration is the usual rule.

Such are the physical changes which have followed in the wake of modern foods. The mental changes have been no less marked. What had been called the world's happiest and most active race has become unhappy, lethargic, and lazy.

Residents and visitors have told in many volumes of the gloom and depression which have settled over these islands. Survivors of the pestilences and diseases see their villages desolated and their friends forever lost.

Missionaries come out to console and save them, but the natives only bring out the deformed and dying and lay them in front of the missionaries, as evidence that the white god does not save them.

The natives see their approaching end. They view it without fear, but with a melancholy and sorrow so tragic and deep that words can hardly describe them. In resigned distress, the people mourn, suffer, and look forward to the inevitable, without confidence and without hope.

"Today," declares O'Brien, "insignificant in numbers, unsung in history, they go to the abode of their dark spirits, calmly and without protest. A race goes out in wretchedness, a race worth saving, a race superb in manhood when the whites came. ...

"Soon none will be left to tell of their departed glories. Their skulls perhaps shall speak to the stranger who comes a few decades hence, of a manly people, once magnificently perfect in body, masters of their sea, unexcelled in the record of humanity in beauty, vigour, and valour."

So concludes the dramatic history of the vanishing Marquesans. Living in their primitive state chiefly upon tropical fruits, plant roots, and coconuts, with moderate amounts of animal sea food, the Marquesans perhaps exceeded all other races in terms of beauty of body, regularity of features, and happiness of mind.

They maintained high immunity to virtually all forms of disease and lived over a great span of years. With the advent of the white man, and the corresponding change in physical environment and dietary habits, the picture rapidly changed, as former qualities and attributes were lost and severe physical deterioration set in. The final tragedy, as is exemplified by modern Marquesan life, stands as a remarkable contrast to the existence of old, when happiness was complete and physical perfection the general rule.

31.

The Pitcairn Islanders

Of the famous sea stories of the past, few compare in drama and excitement with that of the Mutiny on the *Bounty*. The writers, Nordhoff and Hall, have woven the facts and legends of this well-known historical event into the romantic and interesting tale which has been read by millions throughout the world. Later, production on the screen gave many others an insight into the general pattern of this celebrated drama.

The sequel to the story, covering the Pitcairn Island adventure of the seamen who mutinied, has also been told many times.

What has been less often considered, however, and indeed is now almost forgotten, is the experience of the descendants of the mutineers, a little race of its own, which developed a form of primitive nutrition and exemplified a state of primitive health.

The factual data connected therewith has long been available and we shall consider it here, starting with a short introduction which covers very briefly the preceding events of the voyage of the *Bounty* and the associated mutiny.

The story begins in 1787, when HMS *Bounty*, under the command of the notorious Captain William Bligh, sailed from England on a voyage to the South Seas. The ship was fitted out by the English government for the purpose of obtaining plants of the breadfruit tree, which afforded the inhabitants of the Society Islands, in particular Tahiti, a large portion of their nourishment.

This step was taken in response to a request made from the planters and merchants interested in doing business with the government's West Indies. The breadfruit was desired to be transported to these possessions and there planted to serve as a cheap food for the slave labour engaged to work for the English.

The first part of the mission was readily accomplished in the allotted time. Thousands of plants were gathered from Tahiti and placed on board ship. The return voyage was never made, however.

Under the cruel treatment of the brutal Captain Bligh, the majority of seamen mutinied. They placed the Captain and those who remained loyal to him in a small boat at sea, and, taking full control of the ship themselves, they returned again to Tahiti.

Here a number of those on board were left to settle in a new life with the natives. The nine remaining seamen, including Fletcher Christian, the second in command to Bligh, and ten Tahitian women, one girl and six Tahitian men, sailed again in search of an uninhabited island which might afford them a settlement in safety from the punishment of the English government.

Pitcairn Island, located several hundred miles south and west of Tahiti, and not previously visited by voyagers, was chosen, and the landing was made in 1789. Captain Bligh and his party, in the meantime, made their way to the East Indies, landing on the island of Timor after much suffering and hardship at sea.

They were then transferred to England, where they told the story of the mutiny, and action was immediately taken. A ship was sent to Tahiti, where the mutineers who were left were captured.

Four of these died in a shipwreck on the return voyage to England. Of the ten who were tried for mutiny, six were found guilty and four were acquitted. Searches were made in the following years for the *Bounty* and its seamen, but without success.

Returning to Pitcairn Island, we find life beginning successfully for the mutineers, their Tahitian wives and men. Shelters were constructed from the materials at hand; the lands were cultivated, and fish were obtained from the sea. For a few years life was peaceful, and, though there was some quarrelling, co-operation was general pertaining to the necessary work to be done.

Soon, however, there developed jealousy between the men over the affections of the women, and two Tahitian men died mysteriously thereafter, perhaps as a consequence.

Secret plots followed; the remaining Tahitians started a bloody massacre, killing five of the seamen, but in the ensuing battle the Tahitians were also killed, leaving but four men and the eleven women and their children on the island.

The men learned to make a strong liquor from the ti-plant; an orgy of drinking followed, the women sometimes taking part, but later moving elsewhere on the island to live alone and care for their children. Soon, one of the seamen, McCoy, died in a mad suicidal leap from a high cliff. Another, Quintal, was killed by Young and Smith, and the former died of asthma in 1789. Thus, with one seaman, all the women, and by now a flock of children on the island, life proceeded in peace.

Smith taught the children to speak English, also to read, and a primitive community was in the process of development.

The diet of the islanders from the very beginning consisted of the local foods the land and sea could provide. Coconuts, breadfruit, plantains, watermelons, pumpkins, yams, sweet potatoes, taro and sugar cane were in general use. Animal foods were seldom eaten, usually no more often than twice a week, and then consisting of fish or pig. Distilled liquors were not used after the deaths of McCoy and Quintal.

After nineteen years of island life without a visit from the outside world, the American ship, *Topaz*, under the command of Captain Folger, arrived in 1808. Smith came out to meet the ship, along with the others, and he informed the captain of the mutiny and all later experiences.

A chronometer and compass from the *Bounty* were given by Smith for forwarding to the Admiralty, but they were apparently never received in England, for no notice was taken of the discovery until 1814, when HMS *Britain* and *Tagus* arrived under Captains Stains and Pipon. The former related all details of the amazing answer to the *Bounty* riddle to Admiral Dixon, who made them public in England, to the surprise and interest of all.

By this time the little Pitcairn group had multiplied to forty-six, and both captains described the settlement as the happiest and most delightful they had ever seen. Co-operation and contentment were general among all, and the people were very healthy and strong. The descendants of the mutineers were now young men and women of splendid physiques, and their children in turn were also fine in appearance.

Under the wise leadership of Smith, the community prospered in all ways and exemplified all that might be desired. In the words of Captain Stains:

"The young men all born on the island were very athletic, and of the finest forms, their countenance open and pleasing, indicating much benevolence and goodness of heart; but the young women were objects of particular admiration, being tall, robust and beautifully formed, their faces beaming with smiles and unruffled good humour, but wearing a degree of modesty and bashfulness that would do honour to the most virtuous nation on earth;

their teeth like ivory were regular and beautiful; and all of them, both male and female, had the most marked English features.

The clothing of the young females consisted of a piece of linen reaching from the waist to the knees, and generally a sort of mantle thrown over the shoulders, and hanging as low as the ankles, but this covering seemed chiefly as a protection against the sun and weather, as it was frequently laid aside, and then the upper part of the body was entirely exposed, and it is not possible to conceive of more beautiful forms than they exhibited."

Captain Pipon recorded:

"A young girl accompanied us to the boat, carrying on her shoulders as a present, a large basket of yams, over such roads, and on such roads, and down such precipices, as were hardly passable by any creatures except goats, and over which we could scarcely scramble with the help of our hands. Yet with this load on her shoulders, she skipped from rock to rock like a young roe."

The island was again visited a few times during the next decade, and in 1925 the people were host to the illustrious Captain Beechey, who described in detail their happy little settlement, and made the following comments on their health, strength and general agility:

"The Pitcairn Islanders are tall, robust, and healthy. Their average height is five feet ten inches, the tallest person is six feet and one quarter of an inch, and the shortest of the adults is five feet nine inches and one eighth. Their limbs are well proportioned, round and straight; their feet turning a little inwards. The boys promise to be equally as tall as their fathers; one of them whom we measured was, at eight years of age, four feet one inch; and another, at nine years, four feet three inches.

Their simple food and lots of exercise give them a muscular power and activity not often surpassed. It is recorded among the feats of strength which these people occasionally evince, that two of the strongest of the island, George Young and Edward Quintal, have each carried, at one time, without inconvenience, a kedge anchor, two sledge hammers, and an armourer's anvil, amounting to upwards of six hundredweight; and Quintal, at another time, carried a boat twenty-eight feet long.

Their activity on land has been already mentioned. I shall merely give another instance which has been supplied by Lieutenant Belcher, who was admitted to be most active among the officers on board, and who did not consider himself behind hand in such exploits. He offered to accompany one of the natives down a difficult descent, in spite of the warnings of his friend that he was unequal to the task. They, however, commenced the perilous descent, but Mr Belcher was obliged to confess his inability to proceed, whilst his companion, perfectly assured of his own footing, offered him his hand, and undertook to conduct him to the bottom, if he would depend on him for safety.

In the water they are almost as much at home as on land, and can remain nearly a whole day in the sea. They frequently swam round their little island, the circuit of which is at least seven miles. When the sea beats heavily on the island, they have plunged into the breakers and swam to the sea beyond. This they sometimes did pushing a barrel of water before them, when it could be gotten off in no other way, and in this manner we procured several tons of water without a single cask being stoved.

The treatment of their children differs from that of our own country, as the infant is bathed three times a day in cold water, and is sometimes not weaned for three or four years; but as soon as that takes place it is fed upon "Popoe", made with ripe plantains and boiled taro rubbed into a paste. Upon this simple nourishment children are reared to a more healthy state than in other countries, and are free from fevers and other complaints peculiar to the civilised world.

Mr Collie remarks in his journal that nothing is more extraordinary than the uniform good health of the children; the teeth is easily got over, they have no bowel complaints, and are exempt from those contagious diseases which affect children in large communities."

In 1831, it was decided to move the Pitcairn Islanders to Tahiti, and a special ship was provided by the British government for this purpose. On 6th March all left, being given provisions of the usual British seamen's food while on board, and using like foods to some extent after arriving in Tahiti. But little time elapsed before they were taken sick; between 21st April and 21st June, twelve of them passed away. Thus, discontented and fearful for their own lives, the remainder decided to return to Pitcairn Island.

Having chartered an American freighter for this purpose, they left immediately. Three more died, however, before the voyage was ended, and another two died by the end of the year on the island.

The hogs having gone wild and destroyed the crops during the absence from their island, the Pitcairns were still in difficulty, and they took to distilling spirits from the ti-root, many of them drinking to great excess. Fortunately, this was of short duration; in 1833 all stills were destroyed, a law was passed against drunkenness, and all were again feeding upon their native diet. Life had returned to the healthy conditions of the past, and so it was, up to the year 1839, when Lieutenant Lowry visited them and made the following comments:

"At the time of our visit, they had increased to 102 (51 males and 51 females), a great part of them children, and as fine a race as I ever saw. Some of the girls and young women were very pretty, and would be considered beauties in Old England, and all were good looking. There was but one ever born on the island with any defect in his person, and that was only in his eye. Their manner of living is so simple, that they have few diseases, and deaths rarely visit them except in old age."

From here on this story returns to tragedy, as the British took official possession of the island and it became a trading-centre for ships which occasionally stopped. These the islanders provided with sweet potatoes, yams, coconuts, oranges, pumpkins and other items, for which they received tea, flour, biscuits, salt beef, and similar foodstuffs.

The native foods were still used in part, but they were balanced in ever-increasing amounts with whatever importations they might obtain. More than two hundred ships visited the island between 1840 and 1856, leaving provisions of food as the people requested or were able to purchase.

The Register of Pitcairn Island, carefully maintained from 1790 to 1854, as well as accounts from many voyagers, tells of rapid increases of disease taking place from 1841 on. In that year, fifty cases of influenza were reported in a single epidemic. In 1843, the first death from cancer was mentioned, and in the following year sixty of the inhabitants were vaccinated. This seemed only to give the spreading ailments a further impetus, and in 1845 a bilious fever made its appearance, the Register telling us that: "There is not a single house but what there are one or more sick in."

We are also informed in the same year that: "Asthma, rheumatism, consumption, scrofula, and, last but not least, influenza, under various modifications, are prevalent. Five times during the last four years has the fever been rife amongst us, though it has not been so severe lately."

And so the conditions continued. An epidemic in 1849 afflicted every single inhabitant, and it was later followed in many of them by a "most distressing cough". In 1853, influenza returned to render most of the people seriously ill. In 1856, the missionary, Murray, observed that: "Though the climate cannot be called unhealthy, the people are not generally long-lived. Arthur Quintal, the oldest man now among them, is about sixty years old. Elizabeth Young, daughter of the late John Mills, the oldest person on the island, is sixty-four, she having been born in 1792. The ailments to which the people are most afflicted are rheumatism, influenza, bilious affections and diseases of the heart."

The year 1856 marked a closing phase of the Pitcairn Island adventure. As the small area was no longer capable of supporting the increasing population, which now counted 194, all were moved in the British ship *Morayshire* to Norfolk Island, some three thousand miles away. Here life began anew and a permanent settlement was formed. In later years, some of the people again returned to Pitcairn Island. However, in neither area were any important changes made in nutrition, and health conditions remained on the usual level common to civilised society.

Such was the aftermath of the Mutiny on the *Bounty*. Heretofore little known, and then only as a romantic and interesting story, we find it to have serious implications of concern to medicine and nutrition.

From a small group of English seamen, mostly crude sailors, and their Polynesian wives, development of a healthy and happy society, based upon the sound nutritional habits that nature necessitated. From then on, we observe the physical deterioration of the inhabitants of the same settlement, as they gradually lose their isolation and change their mode of nutrition. The experience of these people is one to remember.

It is a lesson to our modern scientists that, instead of searching for cures for this ailment and that ailment, they should instead be looking to restoring our food to a more natural, organic standard, and not be interfering with dietary with heating, processing, irradiation, spraying with toxic chemicals of all sorts, and now, the further insult – Genetically Modified foods! They clearly put money in front of human health.

Looking at these examples of primitive folks, it is clear that no-one – no scientist, no doctor, no physiologist, no biochemist – can improve on nature. These scientists may insist that "science" knows best, but it is clear that the very opposite is true, despite their proclamations that they are making great progress in the search for "cures".

Science suffers from a persistent state of self-deception, as has been stated elsewhere in this book. They might "discover" a new bacterium or micro-organism and claim it is responsible for this illness or that, but what they are finding is the *result* of long-term wrong feeding that *results* in that bacterium or micro-organism existing within that patient suffering from that particular condition.

By simply searching for a drug that will kill that bacterium or micro-organism, they are missing the very reason that bacterium or micro-organism got there in the first place.

168

They will hit a brick wall after brick wall until they realise that, until they focus in on human diet, then they will absolutely *never* find the cause of any illness.

Science has a long way to go, on its present course, to finding answers to overcoming the increasing ill health in our society. And they will only ever find the answer if they abandon the course they are on, realise their folly, and recognise that health will return once people return to a natural way of eating.

The food provided by nature is all we need – without tampering, without interference of any kind. Then, and only then, will human society be free from disease. Scientists earn good salaries and it is their work that gives them a good living. Perhaps the fear that their work will no longer be required as soon as people realise that there is a simple remedy to illness and it involves diet, not science – perhaps it is that which insists scientists keep their heads down and their blindfolds on as to the *true* cause of disease.

32.

Other Island Races

We have considered the above important primitive island races. Now we shall look at others, who have also contributed a significant dietetic and medical history which can be of great use to us today.

These include the remaining Polynesian racial groups, the Melanesians of the New Caledonian and the Fiji Islands, the natives of the Torres Strait Isles north of Australia, the Marianas Islanders, and the inhabitants of Tristan da Cunha in the South Atlantic Ocean.

Beginning with the Polynesian Isles, we view Tahiti, the largest and most famous island of the Society group. Originally it was called one of the most beautiful and delightful of the South Sea Islands. The native population was about 240,000 in number.

Dietary habits were much like those on the Marquesas Islands. Breadfruit was not so abundant, but other fruits and many coconuts and plant roots were plentiful.

For most of the natives these plant foods constituted about nine-tenths of the food supply, the balance being in the form of fish.

Control of the land was in the hands of the superior classes (chiefs, nobles and elders), and they received the choice of plant foods, as well as pig. Food preparation was simple, as among the Marquesans, but there was perhaps more cooking, and fish were consumed both raw and baked.

The first of the European voyagers to see the Tahitians was L. A. Bougainville of France, who arrived at the island on 2nd April, 1768. Bougainville noted the natives to be "free from almost all diseases", being also "better made and better proportioned people" than any he had seen elsewhere. He also observed: "The Tahitians are to be seen bathing in every river that we cross; their vigour and agility, even in old men, surpass those of our young folk. ... The contented old age which they attain, without any infirmities, the acuteness of all their senses and the singular beauty of their teeth – which they keep at the most advanced age – what a testimony to the healthiness of the climate and the wholesomeness of the regimen followed by the inhabitants!"

A few years later, Captain Cook visited Tahiti and his reports of the strength and beauty of the people, and the harmony of their natural life, corresponded with the earlier reports of Bougainville. He stated:

"As to the people, they are of the largest size of Europeans. The men are tall, strong, well-limbed, and finely shaped.

The tallest that we saw was a man upon a neighbouring island, called Huaheine, who measured six feet three inches and a half. The women of superior rank are also in general above our middle stature, but those of the inferior class are rather below it, and rather small. Their natural complexion is that kind of clear olive, or brunette, which many people in Europe prefer to the finest white and red.

In those that are exposed to the wind and sun, it is considerably depended, but in others that live under shelter, especially the superior class of women, it continues its native hue, and the skin is most delicately smooth and soft; they have no tint in their cheeks which we distinguish by colour.

The shape of the face is comely, the cheek-bones are not high, neither are the eyes hollow, nor the brow prominent; the only feature which, in general, does not correspond with our ideas of beauty is the nose, which in general is somewhat flat; but their eyes, especially those of the women, are full of expression, sometimes sparkling with fire, and sometimes melting with softness; their teeth also are, almost without exception, most beautifully even and white, and their breath perfectly without taint."

The Naturalist, Dr Forster, who arrived at Tahiti with Captain Cook, gave the following description of the superior and common people of the island:

"The features of the face were generally regular, soft, and beautiful; the nose something broad below; the chin is overspread and darkened by a fine beard. The women have an open, cheerful countenance; a full, bright and sparkling eye, the face more round than oval; the features heightened and improved by a smile which beggars all description.

The rest of the body above the waist is well proportioned, included in the most beautiful and soft outline; and sometimes extremely feminine. The common people are likewise, in general, well-built and proportioned, but with limbs and joints delicately shaped. The arms, hands and fingers of some are so exquisitely delicate and beautiful that they would do honour to a Venuz de' Medicis."

From the journals of Captain Wilson of the ship *Duff*, we are told that the eyes of the Tahitians "are black and sparkling; their teeth white and even; their skin soft and delicate; their limbs finely turned; their hair jetty, perfumed and ornamented with flowers; they are in general wide and large over the shoulders".

The women "possess eminent feminine graces; their faces are never darkened with a scowl, or covered with a cloud of sullenness or suspicion. Their manners are affable and engaging; their step easy, firm and graceful; their behaviour free and unguarded, always boundless in generosity to each other and to strangers; their tempers mild, gentle, and unaffected; slow to take offence, easily pacified, and seldom retaining resentment or revenge, whatever the provocation they may have received. Their arms and hands are very delicately formed, and, though they go barefoot, their feet are not coarse and spreading."

Similar testimony might be quoted from other voyagers of the 18th century; all indicating much the same, and describing the beauty and general happiness and contentment of the Tahitian people.

Among the superior classes, the luxury of food and the great quantities in which it was consumed often led to a condition of corpulence in later years; but beyond this the people were much as have been described – fine in development, beautiful in features, with teeth of general perfection.

Diseases among them were not common, and the length of life was long, the people retaining strength and vigour into the late years.

Dietary change came gradually at the beginning of the 19th century. The natives were then curiously trying the new foods which the seamen from other lands would bring them. Liquors soon began arriving in quantity, and many made intoxicating drinks from the native ava plant.

Coconut toddy, an intoxicant made from the coconut, also came into widespread use. Coffee, tea, sugar, salt, and tobacco became common items of the new Tahitian life.

Results were quickly forthcoming. Infectious diseases arrived with dramatic suddenness, and by 1850 the great part of the population had died in epidemics of smallpox and tuberculosis, diseases which were unknown before the white man arrived.

Other diseases also became common. In the years 1872-82, Coppinger studied the remaining population and commented as follows upon one aspect of their physical condition:

"A great number of both sexes were affected with a rather unsightly skin disease, evidently of a parasitic character, which they call "pester". It begins on the chest and shoulders in small circular patches somewhat resembling "ringworm", and evidently extends over the entire cutaneous surfaces, causing disfiguration of the cuticle and giving rise to a very distressing itching. When the disease has become well established, the skin exhibits grooves of the "snail-track" pattern, which intersect each other in various distances that on examining at a few distance a man who is extensively diseased, he seems at first sight as if covered with artificial cicatrices, arranged so as to represent some hieroglyphic device. "

Modern studies of the Tahitians indicate continuance of physical deterioration, and a change in mental attitude similar to that seen in the modernised Marquesans. Formerly, the people were lovers of song, dancing, games, and swimming, but these have been forgotten, and all seem depressed and lethargic, as they see their own health fade and the race diminish in number.

A marked narrowing and lengthening of the face, together with decay of teeth and changes in the dental arch form, have all but destroyed the classical Tahitian beauty so highly prized in past generations.

In the First World War, the French moved many of the able-bodied natives to the battlefields of Europe, and most of those who returned were maimed and crippled. Today, less than five percent – only 10,000 – of the original population remain, and nearly all of these are living largely upon refined flour products and canned goods.

Groups still using entirely native foods are very few, but these significantly have escaped all form of physical deterioration, and they are healthy and happy. Those studied by Price were very fine looking, with excellent dental arches and complete immunity to tooth decay.

The next important settlement of the Polynesian race is the Tongan Isles, located south and east of Tahiti, between 18 and 22 degrees South latitude.

The primitive diet here was quite similar to that of other Polynesians. Some of the islands were laid out almost entirely in plantations of breadfruit, coconuts, bananas, plantains, sugar cane, and yams. The superior classes had pig, as well as the choicest of vegetable products, though animal sea foods were available for everyone, and some of the lower order of society included, in small measure, the flesh of rats in their diet.

Captain Cook spoke well of the people, giving these notations in his journal: "They have a good shape, and regular features, and are active, brisk and lively. The women in particular are the merriest creatures I ever met with. ... They have fine eyes, and in general good teeth, even to an advanced age. ... The bodies and limbs of most of the females are well proportioned; and some absolutely perfect models of a beautiful figure."

Captain Cook referred to the presence of a skin disease among some, but, beyond this, stated that he saw "neither sick nor lame amongst them; all appeared healthy, strong and vigorous".

On another occasion he provided similar data, stating that,

"... they may be considered as uncommonly healthy; not a single person being seen, during our entire stay, confined to the house by sickness of any kind.

On the contrary, their strength and activity are in every way answerable to their muscular appearance; and they exert both, in their usual employment and in their diversions, in such a manner, that there can be no doubt of their being as yet little debilitated by the numerous diseases that are the consequence of indolence, and an unnatural method of life."

Few people have been happier in their primitive state than the Tongans. Captain Cook pointed out that "joy and contentment are on every face". The island group was first known as the Friendly Isles, because of the friendly attitude of the natives towards the early navigators. Hundreds of them would throng every new ship that might come, and on shore the visitors would be royally entertained in every manner that was possible.

There were games and dancing almost every day, and swimming and frolicking in the sea were included in the common pastimes.

The Tongan Islands have retained a greater degree of isolation than has any other South Sea group.

During the First World War, the price of copra increased from $40.00 to $400.00 per ton, which brought trading ships with white flour and sugar to exchange for the copra. This was followed by much dental decay and diseases in the port areas; but elsewhere on the islands the people remained generally healthy.

When Price arrived, the trade ships seldom called at the islands, for the price of copra had dropped tenfold and the product was no longer in great demand. The people in the port areas still had dental caries, to the proportion of 33.4 percent, but further decay was arrested and the caries were no longer active. On the more isolated islands, the percentage of dental decay was only 0.6 percent.

The old Hawaiians represent another Polynesian group. About 60 to 75 percent of their calories were derived from the taro root and sweet potato, with coconut, breadfruit, guavas, bananas, papaya, fish, and pig as supplementary foods.

The fish were often eaten raw, though they were highly salted by some of the lower classes, as was the other flesh. Among a few of the chiefs, the ava plant found frequent use.

These islands were discovered by Captain Cook, and, after this great navigator met his death at the hands of natives, Captain King issued the necessary reports.

He stated that the Hawaiians who used great quantities of salt in their diet often suffered from boils and ulcers, and chiefs consuming the intoxicating drinks made from the ava plant suffered severely, having many diseases and being afflicted with early and decrepit old age.

The remaining population, however, constituting the great majority, was described as healthy and happy, fond of running and playing over the sands and disporting themselves for hours in the ocean.

"They seem to have few native diseases among them," declared King. "They are, in general, above the middle size, and well made, they walk very gracefully, run nimbly, and are capable of bearing great fatigue. ... Many of both sexes had fine open countenances, and the women, in particular, had good eyes and teeth, and a sweetness and sensibility of look which rendered them very engaging."

Settlers from Japan and America arrived in the Hawaiian Islands after the discovery, and throughout the 19th century they imported foods for their own use, and for the natives as well. Later came the Chinese, Portuguese and Filipinos, increasing further the food importations.

Finally, the manufacture of canned and refined products was accomplished directly on the islands, and today the native Hawaiian lives primarily on these, adding occasionally a little poi, raw fish, or other native food.

The population of the islands was estimated at about 300,000 at the time of Captain Cook's visit.

Bloody tribal wars during the next score years depleted much of the male population, with an epidemic disease between 1802 and 1807 also killing many thousands. In 1820, missionaries arrived, and three years later they estimated the population at 142,000.

Then came many more traders and considerable business development, and by 1853 the census count indicated only 73,138 natives yet remaining, with measles, whooping cough, diarrhoea and influenza having struck with epidemic force on nearly all islands. Nowadays, there are only a few thousand pure Hawaiians left remaining.

Respiratory ailments and blood vessel diseases now account for the greater proportion of deaths, with severe dental troubles adding to the native difficulty.

According to an early (1934) report of Jones, Larson and Pritchard, covering their Hawaiian investigations, "the teeth of Hawaiian babies of today are often ravaged by decay before they completely erupt. The contour of the face has changed, with a progressive receding of the chin, narrowing of the nostrils and general facial structure, and malformity of the dental arch. From a once proud and noble race, physically sturdy and mentally happy, the Hawaiians have thus deteriorated and suffered, as they now approach possible extinction."

Other Polynesian lands are the Samoan Islands, Phoenix Islands, Cook Islands, and Easter Island. The native experiences here have been much the same as elsewhere. A marked physical decadence has invariably followed the use of imported foods. In American Samoa, this has been most clearly described by many travellers.

The Samoans of centuries past lived chiefly on fruits, coconuts, yams, sugar cane, and many animal sea foods – shellfish, sea crabs, octopus, and bêche-de-mere – most of which were eaten in their raw state.

Their health was then very good; infectious diseases were rare; the people were unusually fertile, and death was said to have resulted in general only from accident or old age.

Today the people are going through the unhappy experiences of epidemics and degenerative diseases. Thompson has described whooping cough and measles as being very common, with yaws afflicting nearly every child, one way or another.

Many of the women are said to be barren. Only in the more remote isolated districts have a few native groups lived almost entirely without modern foods, and they have preserved their normal immunity to disease. Price listed the percentage of dental decay at only 0.3 percent in these sections.

South and east of Samoa lie the Fiji islands, and a few hundred miles beyond these is New Caledonia. Here live members of another race, the Melanesians, a dark people, shorter than the Polynesians, with long, kinky hair and broad, muscular bodies. In their primitive state they were considered very strong and quite healthy, having good physiques and excellent teeth, the latter often stained, however, as a result of chewing the betel nut.

Melanesian foods were fruits, vegetable roots, animal sea food, and pig. Fresh-water fish were used by the natives living near the few mountain streams. Of significance is the fact that treaty arrangements between the warring inland and sea-coast tribes assured an interchange of plants for sea foods at all times, thus assuring both of adequate nutrition.

One of the favourite Melanesian foods was the meat of the coconut crabs. These animals were captured when they climbed the coconut trees to obtain food. They were then placed in large pens and fed shredded coconut until they were so fat that they burst their shells. At this time they were considered delicious and eaten in large amounts.

According to reports in the late 1930s, there were still some Melanesians living on native foods. Physically, they were strong and well-developed, with high immunity to dental caries. The other Melanesians, constituting the great majority, live largely on white-flour products, polished rice, refined sugar, and canned foods.

Their numbers have been decreasing throughout the past hundred and fifty years, and the death rate still exceeds the birth rate. The epidemic diseases have accounted for most of the deaths, with a single epidemic of measles carrying off about 40,000 natives in Fiji in 1875. Today, the degenerative diseases are becoming more common. Dental decay and abscessed teeth are so serious they have been listed as frequent causes of suicide, there being no dentists present in many areas to prevent pain and suffering. General narrowing and lengthening of the face, with crowding of the teeth in the dental arch, have given the modern Melanesian a different appearance than has been characteristic of the race.

In the Torres Strait, between New Guinea and northern Australia, live another dark-skinned people, these of Asiatic and Malay stocks. The numerous small islands in the area each support a population of a few hundred to several thousand. The natives of most of the islands buy their food at government food stores. On the more isolated islands, and even a few on which a number of whites have settled, the native foods are still in use. These include taro, pumpkins, bananas, papayas, and plums as the staple plant foods, together with a great variety of scalefish and shellfish.

The natives of the islands were studied by Price. He found that they suffered from a high degree of dental decay and other disease when foods were purchased from government stores.

The groups using native foods all had "sturdy development throughout their bodies, broad dental arches" and a "close proximity to one hundred percent immunity to dental caries".

The strength of the native swimmers was said to be "almost beyond belief". Dr J. R. Nimmo, a physician on one of the islands, told Price that in thirteen years he had failed to see a single case of malignancy among the four thousand natives using their customary foods. At the same time, he found it necessary to operate in cases of several dozen malignancies among the white population, numbering only a few hundred, all of whom consumed modern foodstuffs. Other conditions requiring surgical interference were also reported to be very rare among the primitive inhabitants.

Next we consider the Marianas Islands, lying about two thousand miles directly east of the Philippines Islands in the Pacific Ocean. When discovered, these islands were represented as a veritable paradise, abounding in everything necessary for life, with delicious fruits – guavas, limes, sweet oranges, breadfruit, bananas, watermelons, etc – found everywhere, and the nearby seas containing great numbers of fish to add to the food supply. The topography was a delightful intermixture of valleys and rolling hills, with clean and well-kept villages to shelter the happy population, then numbering about one hundred and fifty thousand.

The people were of Malayan racial stock, being as dark in colour as those of the East Indies, but taller in stature, more robust and active. Pigaffeta in 1521 referred to the women as being "beautiful and delicate", and other voyagers were likewise complimentary in their comments on the physical appearance of the people. The Marianas were a healthy race; they were naturally cute and ingenious, and, previous to the arrival of the Europeans, they thought themselves to be the only people in the world.

In their disposition they were particularly cheerful; as navigators they were active and intelligent, spending much of their time in the sea, both for pleasure and the acquisition of food.

In 1667, the Spanish missionaries arrived. So zealous were they in the work of converting the natives to Christianity, that soldiers accompanied them for purposes of assistance, and very soon the entire character of native life was changed. Clothing was added; many were made slaves to cultivate the newly-developed rice fields; tobacco was introduced, and the people learned to make cocoa wine from the coconut. Navigation and the sea were forgotten, as nutrition was altered, and a little rice and other food formed a more common daily fare than the fruit and fish of the past.

Commodore Anson relates that, by the time he had arrived at the islands in 1745, some of them had been entirely depopulated by epidemics. Byron, arriving later, noted that many of the islands had become an uninhabitable wilderness, overgrown with impenetrable thickets. Most of the population had died or fled to the Caroline Islands to escape disease and subjection to the Spanish.

Rule was maintained by force of arms, and it made life quite unbearable for the natives. Many women were said to have put an end to their lives by hanging and other ways, some throwing their infants into the sea so they might escape the trouble, disease, and misery of future life.

By the beginning of the 19th century, the work of extermination, or, as the missionaries phrased it, the pacification of the inhabitants, was very nearly completed. The Russian, Otto Von Kotzebue, then arrived in the *Rurick*, and so commented:

"Could I have transported myself back to the time when Magellan discovered these islands, the *Rurick* would long since have been surrounded by many canoes with happy islanders.

This was not the case now; the introduction of the Christian religion has not here diffused its benign blessings, for since that time the whole race of natives has been extirpated. We looked in vain for a canoe or a man on the shore; and it almost seemed that we were off an uninhabited island. The sight of this lovely country deeply affected me. Formerly, these fertile valleys were the abode of a nation who passed their days in tranquil happiness; now, only the beautiful palm trees remained to overshadow their graves; a death-like silence everywhere prevailed."

The same navigator returned to the islands in 1814 and found conditions much the same. Nine-tenths of the remaining population was then concentrated in Guam, we are told, and, according to Shoberl, they were "neither mariners nor swimmers; they have ceased to build boats and are utter strangers to the sea". All their peculiarities and arts, indeed their very language, were lost.

"They live and dress like the Tagalese about Manila, cultivate rice, prepare cocoa wine, chew betel, and smoke tobacco," said Shoberl.

In 1842, about five thousand were left, these all in Guam, of racial intermixture with settlers from Spain, Mexico and the Philippines, all Christians, speaking the Spanish language, and acknowledging no relationship to the original tribes whom they had displaced. Since that time the population has gradually increased, but disease has always remained prevalent, and nutrition is now fully modernised, particularly with respect to the refined starches and sugars of civilisation.

From the Pacific we turn to the South Atlantic and consider very briefly the little island of Tristan da Cunha. The island was once uninhabited, but was settled in the 18th and 19th centuries by settlers from Europe, numbering only a few families. The population rapidly increased, and was eventually a thriving settlement of more than a hundred and fifty people.

Until a few years ago, the sources of food were almost entirely local;

cereals, sugar, tea, and coffee could only be obtained from trade ships, which stopped infrequently, and hence they were rarely used. Potatoes and boiled fish were the staple foods. Milk was occasionally consumed, and at rare intervals a cow or sheep would be slaughtered for food. At nesting season, seabirds' eggs were available, and in the summer and autumn a few vegetables and berries were included in the diet.

Visitors to this island reported the people to be much healthier than those of civilisation, with a higher immunity to disease and a longer duration of life. In 1932, a medical inspection was made of the inhabitants by the surgeon commander of the ship HMS *Carlisle*, which stopped at the island. This revealed that the children were entirely free from rickets, and that such infectious diseases as mumps, measles, scarlet fever, whooping cough, and diphtheria were unknown.

The dental condition of the people was studied by an English physician, Dr Sampson, and later by Dr S. D. Hendricksen, an investigator attached to the Norwegian Scientific Expedition, which visited the island. Both investigators reported the dental arches of the people to be broad, the teeth of regular placement, with high immunity to dental caries. The percentage of decayed teeth, according to Sampson, was only 1.84 percent, and 83.4 percent of the mouths were dentally perfect.

The recent development of the fishing industry in the sea surrounding Tristan da Cunha has brought about a change in the inhabitants' manner of living. A company has been established for the purpose of obtaining and selling large numbers of crayfish, and the company food store supplies the people with various kinds of modern foodstuffs.

A cannery is being constructed, which is expected soon to provide all the islanders with canned foods. The American physician, Dr William Brady, visited Tristan da Cunha in January, 1950, and he reported that the diet of the children had already undergone a significant change, with soft drinks, candy, and white-flour products being consumed. A new medical and dental survey of these people a few years hence might be expected to reveal some interesting and important changes in the general state of public health.

The island races which have been mentioned here represent one of the most important sources of information on the study of primitive man and his food.

The island often gives a degree of isolation not found on the continent, and, so long as this remains, the respective racial groups live upon the food which the land and surrounding sea can provide.

The resulting physical condition of the inhabitants, as we have seen, is generally good, and for some a very high degree of bodily perfection is attained. Yet we see this rapidly disappear under the influence of civilisation, as the dietary habits change in accordance with the importation and manufacture of foodstuffs. The islanders are healthy or sick, as the case may be, in direct ratio to the amount of native or modern foods that are consumed.

It has often been assumed that the reason healthy primitive peoples become unhealthy, soon after the arrival of travellers to their shores, was down to "germs" that the "white man" carried and which the natives had no immunity against.

That is far from the real truth. If anything, the natives had a vastly superior immune system to their visitors; the enormous impact on the natives' health was down to the unnatural foods carried by these travellers and presented to the natives, who would readily consume this new-found "luxury" fare to which they had never before been exposed.

33.

The Madeira-Mamore Railway Workers

Human dietary experiences can be explained in many ways, one of which is the astonishing, but true, case of the men who worked on the railway connecting Bolivia with Brazil.

The Madeira-Mamore Railway Company went into the hands of a receiver in 1914, after constructing a single track two hundred and thirty-two miles long, connecting Bolivia with Brazil.

Alfred W. McCann, in his *Science of Eating*, stated: "The first mile of this railway's objective was to exploit the rubber industry of Southern America, not to advertise the dietetic virtues of ripe fruits, or fruit juices, or the deficiencies of the American diet."

In the construction of its two hundred and thirty-two miles of track, four thousand men were literally starved to death on a diet of white bread. Those who escaped death owed their good fortune to the juice of fruits.

Most of the victims of acidosis, or as they called the disease in the State of Mato Grosso, "beri-beri", are buried in Candelaria Graveyard, three kilometres south of Porto Velho, midway between that town and Santo Antonio – the district explored by Theodore Roosevelt.

When the appalling history of this "poison squad" holocaust was written by engineers connected with the enterprise, all reference to the deaths by white bread among the labourers, after a conference of the railroad officials, was deliberately blotted out.

The officials thought the public might misinterpret the facts at the expense of the country through which the railroad had been projected, and it was decided as a good business policy that no mention should be made of the tragedy in the various articles written for electrical, engineering, and scientific publications.

When P. H. Ashmead, chief engineer of construction, himself a victim of white-bread acidosis, reported on the number of deaths in camp, exception was taken to his figures and his list of four thousand victims was cut in two, so that in the records of the tragedy only two thousand names would appear.

Ashmead, one of the best known consulting engineers of New York, on the day he discovered the first symptoms of his approaching breakdown, determined to take passage for England on the next vessel out. Terrified by what he saw going on about him, he had good reason to fear that he, too, was entering the shadows of death.

The dietetic treatment he finally underwent and which saved him from interment in Candelaria Graveyard, I shall describe.

H. F. Dose, one of the Madeira-Mamore engineers who devoted three years to the completion of the work started by P. H. Ashmead, fortunately made numerous observations and kept in close touch with the twenty doctors in the company. Three of these physicians, among whom was Dr Lucian Smith, were stricken with the disease, but escaped death.

All the facts of the expedition, interpreted under the light of the *Kronprinz Willem* adventure, a poison squad classic that you will soon read of, confirm the instant need of reform.

The labourers, of whom there were originally six thousand, consisted of Russians, Greeks, Turks, Italians, Germans, English, Japanese, Hindus, French, Jamaicans, Barbadians, and Brazilians. The officers, engineers, and doctors were chiefly British and American.

The labourers received the equivalent of $2.40 a day in United States currency. They were charged by the Commissary Department an average of one dollar a day for their food. The cost of this food, its inadequacy considered, was so high that it included the lives of the men.

A half-pound tin of glucose jam was sold to them for one dollar. A No. 2 tin of canned sauerkraut sold for one dollar. A No. 1 tin of canned sausages sold for one dollar. The No. 1 tin contained thirteen ounces. The No. 2 tin contained twenty-seven ounces.

White bread constituted the chief foodstuff of the men. It was baked in the camp from patent flour imported from the United States, in thousand-barrel lots, and was furnished by wholesale grocers in New York City under the most highly advertised brands on the market.

In addition to the white bread were enormous quantities of hard white crackers and tapioca, made from the root of the native cassava plant. Like farina, cream of the wheat, corn flakes, toasties, pearled barley, degerminated corn meal, and polished rice, tapioca is a refined, denatured, demineralised, high-calorie acidifying food.

Supplementing these one-sided units of nutrition were large quantities of lard, coffee, sugar, macaroni, and xarque. A few bags of rice were also included.

In the nature of luxuries, sold to the men at enormous prices, were such foods as canned pork and beans, canned spinach, canned wieners, canned jam, corn flakes, oatmeal and condensed milk. The oatmeal and condensed milk were confined to the officers' quarters.

For breakfast, the labourers ate white crackers and white bread with plenty of black coffee, sweetened with sugar. As they had to pay for their own meals, and pay heavily for them, they economised as much as possible, believing, as most others believed, that bread is the staff of life, and in itself sufficient to maintain strength, energy and health.

At noon, they ate white bread, white crackers and xargue, with more coffee and sugar. Occasionally, dried codfish, ham or bacon was substituted for the xarque. Xarque is dried beef, which looks like leather. It is packed in slabs or layers, weighing fifty pounds each. Each slab is several inches thick, and as dry and hard as wood. Before cooking, the xarque was soaked overnight in water, and then boiled.

In the evening, the men ate more white bread, crackers and xarque, and occasionally indulged themselves in a can of sauerkraut, a can of pork and beans, or a can of jam.

The French, Jamaicans and Barbadians grouped together, and every day made what the others would call "sinkers", a sort of heavy doughnut composed of white flour, sugar, and water, fried in lard.

All of the foods in the labourers' camp, with the exception of the beans, which they ate sparingly on account of their high cost, were of the acid-forming type. The base-forming substances were not only deficient in quantity, they were not present at all.

Acidosis under such conditions was inevitable.

The officers, many of whom escaped serious forms of the disease, enjoyed a larger variety of foodstuffs from which to choose, including dried fruits (base-forming), nuts (base-forming), oatmeal (in itself almost a complete food), and potatoes (also base-forming).

Chief Engineer Ashmead, who ate largely of white bread, mashed potatoes, and fresh meat, obtained by slaughtering in camp an occasional beef-steer imported on the hoof for that purpose, began to manifest the first symptoms of the disease almost as soon as the labourers themselves.

The fresh meat, of which he partook abundantly, and which was reserved for the officers' use, did not act as a prophylaxis against the disease, because fresh meat, or any other kind of meat, lacks the base-forming substances so indispensable to the integrity of the internal secretions.

The first symptoms observed among the labourers and officers affected were manifested in a tendency to stub their toes while walking along smooth roads.

The foot would seem to drag. After that, a slight swelling appeared in the ankles, which gradually extended upwards to the knees, with loss of sensation. When this swelling was at its height, a dent in the flesh made by pressure of the finger would remain for a long time.

Shortness of breath and palpitation of the heart, with tremor of the nerves, were the next symptoms, after which the men began to walk as though they were suffering from locomotor-ataxia, with the halting, hesitating, uncontrolled stride characteristic of that disease.

As the cases advanced, the swelling subsided, and the leg gradually wasted away, until, prior to death, nothing remained apparently but the bone and the skin.

Before death, all the men were completely prostrated and helpless. None of the drugs with which the doctors were provided had any effect. Finally, the doctors ordered "no more rice". They thought that rice was the bugaboo, because they had been reading of the relationship between rice and "beri-beri". They did not know that rice had about as much to do with the fatal outbreak of the disease which they characterised as "beri-beri" as a baby carriage influences the eruption of the molars of its occupant.

As the poor devils gazed in the direction of Candelaria Graveyard, where white flour was to disturb them no more, they might well have chanted, "Eventually! Why not now?"

Chief Engineer Ashmead noticed the development of the disease in his own case under circumstances that impressed all its details upon his mind. The camp had lost a man in the jungle, so dense that once a man got into it he lost all sense of location. When lost, it was a serious problem to find the way back to camp. Ashmead participated in an extended search for the missing man, which failed. As night came on, he gave orders to blow the camp whistle at short intervals until morning, hoping that the sound might give the lost man some guide through the heavy brush.

In directing the search, Ashmead had to climb a slight hill. When he reached the top he was out of breath to such a degree that he had to stop in his tracks. When he removed his leggings that night he thought he noticed for the first time that he was "taking on flesh". He was certainly growing "stouter". His ankles were "thicker".

He soon became sure of this, for, in a few days, he found it difficult to buckle the straps of his leggings. Then came the consciousness that he was losing his appetite for bread and meat. For the first time in his life, he experienced a craving for orange juice. He had never been fond of oranges until that time.

On the fifth day following the first appearance of his ankle symptoms, he noticed that, when he pressed the flesh at the ankle, his finger mark remained.

Labourers were dying around him everywhere. They had "beri-beri", the doctors all agreed. He examined their symptoms and discovered his were like theirs. "I've got it too!" he said, and the doctors ordered him away immediately.

He returned to England and, on the ship, fortunately found plenty of oranges. Throughout the entire journey he ate little else, and, after landing in England, he continued to saturate himself with orange juice. Within sixty days his heart dilatation had disappeared, and, except for a depressing sense of lassitude for the next six months, he was apparently none the worse for his experience.

Ashmead, although he did not know it, was making use of the alkaline earthy salts of the orange to his own benefit.

There was no calcium in the Madeira-Mamore Railway poison squad diet. One of the suppressed facts in connection with its mortality records was the scourge of tuberculosis that swept over the men who escaped "beri-beri".

Both Ashmead and Dose confirmed that they lost as many men through tuberculosis as through the disease the doctors knew as beri-beri. All other engineering enterprises, all other large contracting efforts, all other army or navy expeditions or exploring adventures in which, through accident or ignorance, the base-forming elements of food are not properly provided, meet with the same fate.

The chief base-forming foods are oranges, lemons, and ripe fruits of all kinds, the outer grains, such as whole wheat, whole corn, natural brown rice, whole rye, greens of all kinds, lettuce, beet tops, celery, spinach, cabbage, onions, cauliflower, asparagus, the roots of tubers, potatoes, carrots, parsnips, turnips, beets, beans, peas, lentils, nuts of every kind and unsulphured dried fruits, such as prunes, black raisins, currants, sun-dried apples, apricots, and peaches.

So many people in our modern world suffer from malnutrition without knowing it. From anaemia, from impaired vitality, from lowered resistance to disease, from "laziness", and from other serious departures from normal physical stamina that end in misery, impaired efficiency, and untimely death, that it is time indeed the public understood the relationship between base-forming and acid-forming foods.

The deaths of the four thousand railway labourers who built those two hundred and thirty-two miles of railway that run by the Candelaria Graveyard represent not only preventable loss of life, due to ignorance of the laws of nutrition – not only of the men, but of the company's doctors – but they also represent tremendous financial losses sustained by the builders of the railway who, handicapped by sickness and inefficiency, poured more money into the construction of their project – a hundredfold more – than would have been necessary had the diet of their men been properly safeguarded and less false economy invoked.

It is a curious but tragic fact that thousands of healthy monkeys played around the Madeira-Mamore camp where human beings were dying in their thousands. The monkeys lived, enjoyed life, and maintained their energy and activity on a diet of tropical fruits and nuts. Their presence in the vicinity of the sick labourers, who fell as fast as they might fall in battle, seemed to be an effort of Mother Nature to speak to her unfortunate human children, suggesting a remedy was at hand for their misery.

The food of the monkeys was available. It was base-forming food; but the men, who, even as labourers, had conceived astonishing ideas of class distinction, had already dubbed it "monkey food". In their reluctance to subsist on "monkey food", they rejected what would have saved them.

It will probably not go unnoticed to the reader that even today we have sufferers with shortness of breath, puffy ankles, etc, which are similar to these labourers. Beri-beri is seen as a vitamin B1 deficiency, common in alcoholics. My own aunt had the swollen ankles, breathlessness, and heart problems, when I told her about the possibility it could be her diet. She persevered with a diet I gave her – rich in fruits and salads, and, within a couple of weeks, her lower legs were almost completely normal – something her own doctor had failed to do all the time he was prescribing water tablets and medication for her heart.

It has been stated that someone could walk into a doctor's surgery presenting with all the symptoms of beri-beri, and, even now in 2012, the doctor would be completely unaware that the cause was of a dietary nature.

An example I use is: if someone was foolish enough to live on, say, jelly babies (or candy in America), for, say, a full year, the chances are that person – assuming he was still alive – would have fatigue, perhaps bad skin, and depression.

If he went to his doctor's presenting with these symptoms, chances are very high that he would walk out of the surgery clutching a prescription for some drug or ointment for his skin, a drug for his depression, and medication for his fatigue. The doctor will have completely missed the *cause* of the patient's illness, simply because he has received no training in this area – something that will never change as long as colossal profits exist for the drug industry.

34.

Value of Primitive Foods

Good health in the primitive world is related to the naturalness of their native nutrition. As their native food is replaced by the typical civilised dietary regimen, we observe immediate deterioration, both physical and mental.

Practically every form of previous immunity is lost. Bacterial scourges arrive first, the degenerative diseases become common later. For the majority of races, the population rapidly diminishes in number as the first consequence.

This may continue for decades or centuries, until extinction, or until a stabilising point is reached, when the birth rate again gradually increases and the death rate falls. The race again becomes prolific, with an increase in numbers, but with continuing disease and ill health, as is typical in the average civilised community.

What, therefore, are the qualities or factors found in native primitive foods which have been successful in sustaining a high degree of physical excellence? Also, what are the qualities or factors found in modern foods which have failed on all counts to meet the necessary requirements? How are we to account for the very great differences involved?

A detailed answer would require volumes to explain. A limited answer, sufficient for the purposes of this book, will briefly cover the most important nutritional concepts involved, and it may be sufficient to allow a practical understanding and application of these to our modern life.

Biologically speaking, the human body is a chemical and physiological unit, depending for its efficiency of function upon the many nutritional elements – known and yet to be discovered – found in our food. You must also realise that there will be complex crossover influences amongst all these nutrients, about which it would be virtually impossible to fully understand.

A natural food, raw and unrefined, grown in fertile soil and consumed in its fresh state, contains maximum amounts of the chemical elements needed by the human body. Its physical state is such as to permit proper digestion and assimilation. As a part of the normal nutriment for animal life, it is generally adequate, the recipient species living in a condition of excellent health, with usual freedom from disease.

As the food is altered, it becomes less complete as a nutritional unit. Separating the food in to fractions, as in the process of refining – discarding certain of the fractions and consuming others – means that a number of nutritional qualities will be lost. Heating the food at high temperatures is likewise associated with nutritional losses and changes in physical structure.

Other forms of processing and treatment – the addition to the food of various irritants and synthetic ingredients, and then prolonged storage – all these tend to detract from the original value of the food. In a condition of undisturbed nature there are no such practises of food interference.

The same is true of the fruits and plants grown in virgin soil. One could scarcely find a greater contrast than the health and vigour of the average wild plant, and the susceptibility to disease of the usual cultivated plant grown in commercially treated soils.

The former, growing in the rich and undisturbed lands of high organic content, is highly nutritious, and, because of its natural immunity, does not attract parasites. This is in sharp contrast to commercial plants, which can be susceptible to parasite attacks. Parasites, it has been noted by farmers, do not attack healthy plants, only the unhealthy.

For many primitive groups, the predominant or entire portion of plant food is obtained in the wild state from the fertile soils of forests and plains. In civilisation, the opposite is true; scarcely any wild fruits or plants are included in the typical dietary regimen.

Animals living on nutritious plant life may be expected to yield more nutritious flesh than animals fed in the usual modern manner. The primitive gets his flesh from healthy wild animals or domestic animals which are properly fed and cared for.

Quality, not quantity, is the primary object. This is contrasted to civilisation, where domestic animals are fed in a manner deliberately calculated to produce an abnormal amount of fat or meat.

An excellent example is to be found in the case of the domestic hog. In civilisation, the animals are carelessly fed practically all edible substances, including garbage and slaughter-house wastes, in many cases coming to market with a parasitic infection.

The primitive Polynesian and other racial groups of the South Sea Islands raised hogs which were free from such parasites. The animals were fed on an exclusive diet of breadfruit, coconut, taro, and yams. They were much cleaner than American and European hogs; they were not allowed to scavenge, and did not have the habit of wallowing in the mire. According to Forster, the flesh of such animals was of superior quality: "the fat was to be compared to marrow, and the lean had the tender taste of veal".

Porter noted that it was "remarkably sweet and delicate", and Melville described it as "the most docile and amiable pork" which "possesses a most excellent flavour".

Healthier animals also mean better eggs and milk. The egg yolk has long been considered a rich source of vitamins, but it is known that the vitamin content is seriously affected by the food eaten by the hen.

So, too, with milk. The nutritional value of the milk depends on the health of the cow, and the health of the cow depends on the food that the cow eats. The health of the food itself that the cow eats depends on the state and nutritional status of the soil – the least interfered with, the better; the more natural, the superior the health of the soil.

The nutritional content of cow feed is very high when the animal is living on richly-coloured grasses which contain all the vitamins, minerals, and other nutrients, in abundance.

The milk of the dry-fed animal is often so deficient in fat-soluble vitamins that it is inadequate even for the ration of the calf. Its nutritional value is generally no higher than that of ordinary pasteurised milk.

The primitive judges his cattle by the amount of time it takes for a new-born calf to get up and run. This, as is the case with reindeer and many other herbivorous animals, is but a few minutes in most cases.

In civilised society, where quantity of milk and butter fat is the sole object, many of the calves are not able to stand for many hours, often as long as twenty-four.

The difference lies in the feeding of the animals – less dry feed and more rapid-growing green grass, sunshine, and exercise for cattle of the primitive. All cheese is made in the summer, after a heavy period of green-feeding, when the mineral and vitamin content of the milk and cream is at its highest. Price found that in Loetschental Valley the dairy products had a much higher vitamin content than is average throughout the world. Even the stored green hay of the area was comparatively high in chlorophyll.

In the choice of animal foods, the primitive is likewise at an advantage. Instead of restricting his choice of flesh chiefly to muscle meat, which is the least nutritious of all animal parts, he is usually a whole-carcass eater, consuming all edible parts of his quarry. The vital organs are given particular preference, and these are of high nutritional value.

The Indians of northern Canada make a special effort to include in their diet the adrenal glands and walls of the second stomach of all the moose they kill. The Eskimo prefers certain layers of skin in one of the species of whale.

It is known that these animal parts are extremely rich in vitamin C, and thus are important for preventing scurvy, which otherwise might develop on a near-carnivorous diet. Many primitives also make it a point to consume the eyes of all fish, along with the tissues immediately at the back of the eyes. Recent nutritional inquiry indicates that these are of exceptional value; the eye retina and the tissues mentioned are among the richest of all animal sources in vitamin A content. The marrow of animal bones, so preferred by the primitive, adds as well to the supply of fat-soluble vitamins.

Another difference between civilised and primitive dietaries is the feeding of infants.

In civilisation, breast-feeding is rarely employed for more than a few months, if it is employed at all. Yet its importance may be gauged by the experience of the Infant Welfare Centre of Chicago in the years 1924-25, when 20,161 infants were cared for. Of these, 9,794 were wholly breast-fed, 8,605 were partially breast-fed, and 1,707 were artificially-fed.

The mortality rate of the last group was fully fifty-six times greater than among the breast-fed infants, and the rate among those partially breast-fed was four times as high. The difference was accounted for in part by the deaths resulting from respiratory infection, and, to a lesser degree, gastro-intestinal ailments. Whereas only four of the breast-fed infants died of respiratory infections, eighty-two of the artificially-fed infants died from this cause.

That experience can explain the superb health of the normal primitive infant.

The fact is that virtually every primitive infant is breast fed, and the nursing period extends in most cases from two to three years, the mother's milk being the basic food during that time. If the supply fails, which is not often, the infant is usually nursed by another lactating woman.

Among island races with no cattle, survival itself is dependent upon the long nursing period. Whilst dairying races are able to use animal milk if required, it is seldom done for infant feeding, preferring instead the mother's milk.

The general primitive choice of foods in an isolated environment rarely permits the use of salt, spices, and similar substances which, as shown both by human observation and animal experiment, impair physiological efficiency and are irritating to tissues. Similarly, tea and coffee are never to be found in the primitive diet.

Of equal interest is the freshness of primitive food. Nutritional losses as a consequence of preservation are not experienced. Grains are made into bread on the same day that they are ground. Fruits are often sun-dried, but beyond this are rarely treated for preservation. Animal flesh is usually consumed raw – immediately after the animal is killed.

There are exceptions, which have been mentioned, with respect to the less favourable primitive groups, and these are associated with signs of physical inferiority not generally found elsewhere.

Important is the fact that none of the primitive foods is refined. In the manufacture of white flour, an average of four-fifths of all minerals and vitamins are lost. Regarding refined sugar, the losses are even greater.

The most important nutrients of rice, as in wheat, are in the outer hull, which is discarded during the refining process. In the average modern diet, up to 25 percent of all calories are taken in the form of sugar, and over half of the diet is composed of products made from refined sugars and starches. The primitive, getting no such foods, escapes the most important single cause of nutritional deficiency.

No primitive foods are canned. This is very important, considering the fact that many minerals and vitamins are lost in the canning process. This is due in part to the greater or longer application of heat than is usual in ordinary cooking. There are also further nutritional losses while the food remains in storage.

The addition of salt and refined sugar to many canned foods adds to the general impairment of the product.

On an average, cooking is less often employed by the superior primitive races than it is by either the inferior primitive races or civilised man. Losses of minerals and vitamins, and destruction of necessary cellulose in plant foods, are thus reduced. All milk and milk products are used in their raw state, pasteurisation being unknown. In many cases, even the animal flesh or sea food is eaten in its raw state.

Such foods that are cooked usually undergo exposure to heat for a shorter period of time than is customary in civilisation, and where there is cooking water it is served with the foods, thus providing the consumer with the valuable water-soluble minerals.

The Hunzas of India, for instance, cook their whole-grain chapatis for a mere few seconds before twitching them off to a platter for later consumption.

Among the Polynesians and other races of the South Sea area, the process of enclosing food in banana or palm leaves and placing this on the red-hot stones of underground ovens, then covering it all with a generous supply of earth, is the least destructive of all methods of cooking. The earth keeps the steam from escaping, and the food thus loses a minimum of flavour and nutritional elements. Actual losses in minerals and vitamins do not exceed one third of those resulting from modern cooking procedures involving the boiling of foods in water.

The advantages of primitive foods thus range from soil to choice and the methods of preparation. Just how important these are may be understood from the work of Price.

In his travel in all parts of the earth, this scientist obtained samples of every food used by each primitive group he visited. These were subjected to chemical analysis for their mineral and vitamin content, and then compared in this respect to the common foods of civilisation.

The results indicated that the typical primitive diet was several times as rich in the necessary nutritional factors as is the typical modern diet. Exact figures were given in regard to some of the minerals, and these are given here, together with data on the fat-soluble vitamins, in tabular form.

The numbers in the various columns show how many times as much of the respective elements are found in the respective primitive diets as in the modern diet. For instance, the table shows that the diet of the Australian Aborigine contains 4.6 times as much calcium, 17 times as much magnesium, 50.6 times as much iron, 6.2 times as much phosphorous, and 10 times the amount of fat-soluble vitamins as in the modern (displacing) diet. The rest of the table may be read accordingly.

Race	Calcium	Magnesium	Iron	Phosphorous	Fat-Soluble Vitamins
Australian Aborigine	4.6	17	50.6	6.2	10
New Zealand Maoris	6.2	23.4	58.3	6.9	10
Melanesians	5.7	24.4	22.4	6.4	10
Polynesians	5.6	28.5	18.6	7.2	10
Cattle tribes of Interior Africa	7.5	19.1	16	8.2	10
Agricultural tribes of Interior Africa	3.5	5.4	16.6	4.1	10
Eskimos	5.4	7.9	5.5	5	10
Indians of Northern Canada	5.8	4.3	2.7	5.8	10

Coastal Peruvian Indians	6.6	13.6	5.1	5.5	10
Peruvian Indians of the Andes	5	13.3	29.3	5.5	10
Native Swiss	3.7	2.5	3.1	2.2	10
Gaelics	2.1	1.3	1.0	2.3	10

The ten-fold ratio for fat-soluble vitamins was listed by Price as the minimum for the respective racial groups, though in some instances it was in excess of this figure. In all of the primitive diets there was a large increase in the amount of water-soluble vitamins over those of the displacing diets. Iodine amounts were also listed for Indian and Eskimo diets, these being 8.8 and 49 times as great as in the displacing diets.

Clearly, primitive nutrition is superior to modern nutrition, despite all the apparent "advances" of science. In supplying many times the quantity of nutritional factors as the latter, it indicates an important approach to the optimum standards of nourishment which are normal to animal life in a condition of nature.

This is significant in terms of possible application to civilisation. If we are to benefit from the primitive experiences, we must adopt the better features of primitive nutrition in our own dietary programmes.

Briefly, the changes required would be:

1. Rational methods of soil care (no spraying with chemicals). In other words, organic.
2. Proper feeding of domestic food animals (no artificial pellets or other refined feed).
3. Abstinence from irritating, stimulating and intoxicating foods and beverages.
4. Abstinence from canned foods and all tinned and processed meats.
5. Discontinuance of pasteurisation of dairy products.
6. Reduction of cooking process, in time and temperature, to minimum. Preferably none.
7. Breast feeding of infants in all cases, but dependent upon diet and health of mother.
8. Consumption of fresh foods, in their raw state, eaten as soon as possible after gathering.
9. Consumption of whole grains and whole-grain products instead of (white flour) refined foods.
10. Use of honey or other natural sweetening agents instead of white sugar.

11. Liberal consumption of fruits, vegetables, nuts, and other foods in their raw state.
12. Arrangement of diet in such a manner as to ensure maximum variety of all healthful foods.

The story of primitive man and his food is an important one. By eating as nature intended – by eating foods in their natural state – we may expect to experience a degree of health, mental as well as physical, which was common amongst these native peoples, but which is so lacking today in our modern societies.

35.

Mental Illness and Violence: The Food Connection

Dr George Watson, in his 1972 book, *Nutrition and Your Mind*, told the case of a lady who had suffered from depression for decades; who had spent thousands of dollars on psychiatrists and an untold number of hours on the couch, and was no better. When tested for food allergies, her depression was immediately shown to be related to a dietary factor and from then on she was in control of her illness. She had at last found a "tool" by which she could finally control her debilitating condition.

That scenario is commonplace. And has been since the food "allergy" connection to illness was made. Allergy groups have sprung up all over the world, with patients taking the condition into their own hands after their collective doctors denied the syndrome even existed.

Even today, over half a century later, doctors still deny the existence of the possibility that ordinary foods can trigger illness, despite the phenomenon being well known in the alternative medicine world. My own research into it earlier in the book shows that there is a blood flow reduction within the body when the food or drink is consumed.

The fact that the brain should be involved should not surprise anyone with intelligence.

The workings of the brain have been shrouded in mystery for centuries and there is no doubt at all that the impossibly complex workings of the brain would defy any man; any scientist.

However, the food that you eat is reduced within the body and carried by the bloodstream to every part, including the brain. This mysterious organ is not exempt from the journey of the blood. All areas of the brain are bathed in this life-giving fluid.

Whilst medical training insists on specialists for various organs of the body – for example, a psychiatrist for the brain; an endocrinologist for the endocrine system; a cardiologist for the heart, and a haematologist for disorders for the blood – the truth is, the health of all these parts is governed by the one event – what you eat.

It is all the more telling that they are connected by the fact that when people do change their diet to one that is natural, omitting all the contrived and artificial foods and instead feeding off foods as close to their natural state as possible, given time, all their illnesses will go away. If the patient has psoriasis, for example, that patient's skin condition will be restored to health (see chapter on Psoriasis), and, if the new method of eating is sustained, then older, familiar problems – for example, warts or lack of energy or any other problem – will also resolve itself.

It is merely a matter of mechanics. If there are blockages in the blood flow anywhere in your body, then the blood and its nutrients are not gaining full access to that part which is blocked, resulting in disorders beyond the blockage.

Such blockages will have been caused by plaque in your blood vessels, built up over years of eating foods that have been cooked or simply deficient in nutrients. Cooking destroys the enzymes in the very food that you are eating; the enzymes which are there to enable the body to use such foods.

If there is a build-up of plaque in a blood vessel, then, by eating a diet rich in natural foods filled with nutrients, that new wave of nutrient-filled blood will wash through your body, slowly and surely eroding away the plaque in your blood vessels.

Because the original plaque will be the oldest – and the hardest – it will take longer to be removed than the relatively recent deposits.

You will find, therefore, that the older conditions in your body will take longer to fully recover from, as opposed to the relatively newer ones.

This is well known in Nature Cure and is called "re-tracing".

As Charlote Gerson, daughter of Dr Max Gerson, would often point out, "the body does not just heal one condition, but, if allowed the time, will heal all that is wrong with the body".

The longer you continue on a natural diet, the more your problems will dissolve away, one by one.

I remember once explaining this to my doctor, and the incredulity that washed over her face was priceless. She must have thought I was daft, but I just knew she was ill-informed in the subject. After all, I had been studying it for over 30 years by that time – she had studied it only for the 30 seconds of time it took for me to put that suggestion to her!

Those doctors who *do* take Nature Cure on board very often wholeheartedly embrace it as being thoroughly logical, and, indeed, commonsensical. There have been many notable physicians down the past hundred or so years who have done just that: Dr George Clements, Dr Max Gerson, and hundreds, if not thousands, of others.

Returning to the issue of mental illness. ... The brain is just yet another part of the body, fed by the same bloodstream that feeds the fingernails, or the knee joints, or the thyroid glands.

People have asked in the past: how can food directly affect the brain, and, indeed, the mental functioning of the entire human body?

It is harder for a medical doctor to readily accept this fact because he has been trained in a different way to those involved in natural healing.

But where does a psychiatrist ask you to put an anti-depressant tablet, so that it changes the function of your brain? IN YOUR MOUTH. The same place as you put your food. The connection cannot be clearer.

Yet again, it is the duty of this book to warn you that if you have a mental illness, you should **not** reduce or stop any medication your doctor has prescribed for you, as this could be very dangerous.

Rather, you should seek out a naturopath, or a natural hygienist, or a nature cure specialist, who have experience in the treatment of people with psychiatric or mental disorders.

Whether it is a full-blown psychopathic disorder or a mere mild anxiety, both could be brought about by unnatural feeding. The Pottenger Cats study is a simple examination of how feeding an animal a cooked diet can result in the cats attacking their keepers and fighting with each other. The cats which were fed a natural, uncooked, raw diet had no such problems.

That is a simple example, but a very pertinent one, of how wrong eating can affect the behaviour of a cat – in that instance – but also because humans are also animals that eat food; the likelihood that eating unnatural (cooked) food should not be lightly dismissed.

At the beginning of this chapter, I mentioned the lady with depression and her discovery that she had food "allergies" and that she could then control her illness.

Finding your food "allergens" is one thing, but being able to totally remove the entire depressive state altogether should be the target. Most people who advertise themselves as able to identify your "food allergies" are only going some of the way and not fully advising the patient that there is yet further to go.

Identifying those triggers is good. It gives you a degree of control over your mood swings that wasn't there before.

Mood swings are famously "food allergic" in origin. Have you ever wondered why someone can "change" for no apparent reason – whether adult or child? Chances are high that there is a dietary component and no-one is advising them of it.

It is all very well trying to treat a child with such problems with behavioural therapy; it is good as far as it goes, but you would be missing a critical aspect of the child's condition that seems to be less known now than when it was first promulgated in the 1960s.

Do not underestimate the powerful effect of food allergies. A simple food can turn a mild-mannered child into a monster within an hour, baffling the long-suffering mother who may well be at her wits' end. The mere instruction on how to identify a dietary component would have been all she needed. But she certainly would *not* get that from her family doctor. ...

Basil Shackleton, who wrote one of the two books entitled *The Grape Cure* (the other author was Johanna Brandt, with a book of the same title), went on that mono diet for a reason – an abscess in his one remaining kidney; his other kidney was removed in his earlier years.

His observation that he changed from an irascible man, irritated at the smallest thing, to someone who "didn't know how to get angry" was an indication of how the bloodstream can be cleansed by consuming clean, natural, pure foods – such as the grape.

Perhaps if all of us were to change to a natural diet or raw foods, we would all be better tempered with pleasant personalities – *along with* freedom from disease. Like the Marquesa Islanders, like the Hunzas, and other primitive – but happy and healthy – tribes.

Your body will heal itself, given the chance. Given natural, clean, unadulterated food, the body's nutritional status will be elevated and the body, being a self-cleansing mechanism, will remove all former rubbish accumulated in the tissues and cells. This may take some time, and the longer you have had your condition, the longer it may be before it is resolved. But, be aware that there are two factors that are important in your recovery: the right food, and time. Given both, and health can be restored.

It is all the more tricky to convey this principle to someone who may have an anxiety condition, because, when someone is in that state, it is very difficult to rationalise with them, especially something so "bizarre" as the fact that, by doing something (they think) they have been doing all their lives, suddenly they are going to get well.

By suggesting that, by eating differently, their "mental" condition can be removed, must seem like the suggestion of a mad man to anyone in a state of neurosis or extreme depression. And all the more so when it doesn't work within hours, or overnight. It takes time to recover – weeks or months – but improvement can be seen sometimes after a mere 4 or 5 days.

The (very) happy compromise of tracking down food allergens is the first move, the identification of foods responsible for the symptoms. Or drinks, or inhalants – anything taken into the body can be the culprit.

There are numerous ways to identify food allergens, and many – like blood tests – are simply not reliable. You may pay hundreds of pounds or dollars for a test, and such expense may suggest you are getting value for money, but if you read my chapter on food allergies you will see that the result of this award-winning and original and unique research is that there can be micro-organisms within your system that feed off your own foods or drinks; then, by dint of such feeding, they can swell up and block or partially block the blood vessel in which they are residing.

Therefore, the blood tests or hair tests for allergens do not address this issue. The real test would be to take the micro-organisms out of the body and individually feed them, in a laboratory, to see which foods they like and which they don't. An impossible and even ridiculous task, but it would be the only way of truly testing. Blood tests – by sending a sample of your blood to be tested – can never hope to achieve the same answers. They would be testing the blood cells for a response, when they should really be testing the *micro-organisms*.

There are many tests for food allergies: blood tests, hair sample tests, and others. They are only good for producing "good" and "bad" reactions to foods. But following such "good" or "bad" food lists does in no way guarantee that you will find the foods responsible for your condition.

I recall sending away for blood tests for myself many, many years ago, and when I received the list of foods to avoid and foods I could freely eat, they were all mixed up from my own knowledge as to what I was allergic to, which I already knew. Potatoes, which I had clearly identified as causing me problems, appeared in the *safe* list – and there were several other anomalies. The laboratory to whom I complained agreed they could not identify every culprit food. I asked how accurate their testing was and they replied 90 percent. I asked them if they would be good enough to tell me the 10 percent that was not accurate so I could work it out myself. They couldn't, unsurprisingly.

Any testing method can come up with a list of foods to avoid and a list to eat freely. But be warned that you simply *cannot* rely on these results. Many people get such tests carried out, use the information as gospel, so to speak, and live the rest of their lives eating foods that still cause them problems.

The only **real** answer is to completely change your diet to a natural, raw one, for, say, three months, just to see the result. Chances are, you will see a huge difference in your health and that will inspire you to continue beyond that experimental period of twelve weeks!

But to immediately put the reader into a sense of checking for food allergies, you should not, once you get up in the morning, smoke or drink any artificial drinks, except water. Then it would be no bad thing to even avoid breakfast – if you commonly experience symptoms in the late mornings. The breakfast that you have been eating for years could – and I only say could – be responsible for a change in your symptoms, mental or physical.

By not eating your breakfast, and, hopefully, being relatively clear of symptoms, up until lunchtime, then your symptoms aggravated in the early to mid-afternoon could be an indication that your lunch was responsible for the change in your mood.

It is best to keep a food diary, putting in absolutely *everything* that you eat or drink, and at what time. Then, also mark in your diary any symptoms you get, again with the time, and how long the symptoms last (and what, if anything, you consume during the duration of these symptoms).

If you keep the diary, it is best not to fill in the list of foods you eat after your meal. It is best to write down the ingredients on the plate before you start eating. If you leave it to when you have finished, you might miss out that mushroom or the watercress that you had forgotten about.

It can be devilishly deceptive working out the foods that can cause you problems.

I remember, during the early years of my trying to work out what foods caused me problems, being absolutely *certain* eggs were responsible for a sudden depression that I would get. I would regularly eat a boiled egg sandwich at a nearby cafe and, about an hour or so later, used to have my hated symptoms come on like clockwork! I used to stand outside before going in and, using positive thinking, say to myself that it will not happen this time; that I simply will *not* let it happen.

As admirable as that might have been, it never worked – I would always suffer as a consequence of eating that egg sandwich! I avoided eggs whenever I could as a consequence.

However, about ten years later, I decided to do something I had avoided for a long time. To eat nothing for a day, then individually test one food at a time. A most time-consuming and frustrating method, but one which could serve you well.

Remember, this was before I knew the simplest answer of all – just stop cooking your food and revert to eating like Man was intended to eat – raw – and thereby build up health within your body and clear out your system.

I was testing one food at a time and watching for symptoms. One morning I tested watercress and went out about my business as normal. I had deliberately eaten a real load of watercress, so that any reaction would be clear cut and without doubt.

About an hour or so later, I had a *tremendous* reaction to it. As that was the only food I had consumed, and I had drunk nothing at all that morning, and inhaled nothing of consequence, the watercress had to be the guilty food.

Not only that, but the reaction lasted an astonishing *six hours*!

Later that day, when I was recovering from the reaction and considering what had happened, a sudden realisation came across me that changed my entire approach to the whole thinking about food detection.

The egg sandwiches that I so loved, but which symptoms that were brought on I reviled, because of the egg reaction, was not about the eggs at all! I had gone years avoiding them whenever possible, thinking they were responsible for my symptoms. But it turned out it was the *watercress* that was IN the egg sandwiches which was doing the damage!

Now, that had passed me by, that simple connection, for a decade. It was an incredible eye-opener, but it shows you that even when you "know" what you're doing, as I prided myself on being able to, there can still be surprises and twists along the way.

Many groups set up by parents offer advice. Many, however, have not got the full grasp of the situation – that the child's complete diet needs to be changed to a natural one. What they do, instead, is focus on sugar in the diet, additives in the diet, chemicals in the diet, salicylates in the diet, monosodium glutamate, and so on. They all purport to know that it might be this, or it might be that, which is responsible for your child's hyperactivity or being withdrawn.

In my own testing at the Royal Infirmary of Edinburgh, I took organic grape juice with me, to take after my first blood flow test (when I had had nothing to eat or drink). Immediately after the all-clear, I consumed a goodly amount of the grape juice in that clinic and waited for the radiologist to return from his duties to re-test me. When he did, he was astonished that my *prediction* that a reduced blood flow would occur on the after-food test had come true. He was not happy that I had beaten him to a discovery in the very field in which he was expert, but nevertheless he was astonished. But I was not. I was happy because it confirmed my long-time thinking on the issue.

But the point I make is that it was organic grape juice that brought about the reaction! Not additives, not chemicals, not E numbers, not preservatives – as many self-help groups focus on.

You may well ask: how can a truly natural food such as organic grape juice bring about a reaction, when this very book is all about eating natural?

The only reasonable offering is that the micro-organisms are already in the body. They may well consume anything that comes in, preferring some foods to others. As that was my first food of the day, that could well have stimulated them into action.

However, that was the very, very short term. Once you have removed ALL cooked and processed food from your diet, you will change the "internal environment" of your body, so that the gases in the bloodstream that are brought about by what you eat, and what the micro-organisms are attracted to, alter completely and become obnoxious to any parasite.

Remember that any farmer will tell you that parasites only attack unhealthy plants; they do not affect healthy ones. That same approach can be applied to humans. Change your diet to become healthy, and parasitic micro-organisms will stay clear of you.

In my case – and probably that of most food allergics – I had a low body temperature. By eating natural foods, my body temperature ever so slowly increased. This raising of the body temperature proves too much for micro-organisms, which are almost certainly attracted to the lower body temperature and filthy internal environment that attracted them to colonise your system in the first place.

Mental illnesses of many kinds can be overcome by sustaining a natural diet. But certainly, if you have a history of taking medication for your symptoms, you need help in coming off them; in which case you should be monitored by your doctor. Approaching a naturopath skilled in this area initially, or a Nature Cure practitioner to get their advice would be a good idea, but you do need your doctor's regular assessment in case of severe reactions.

Regarding children's behaviour, this was reported in 1999:

"In a new review of two dozen scientific studies, the non-profit Center for Science in the Public Interest (CSPI) contends that food dyes and certain foods can adversely affect children's behavior. CSPI, in a 32-page report titled "Diet, ADHD, and Behavior," charges that federal agencies, professional organizations, and the food industry ignore the growing evidence that diet affects behavior.

The report cites 17 controlled studies that found that diet adversely affects some children's behavior, sometimes dramatically. Most of the studies focused on artificial colors, while some also examined the effects of milk, corn, and other common foods. The percentage of children who were affected by diet and the magnitude of the effect varied widely among the studies. Six other studies did not detect any behavioral effect of diet.

It makes a lot more sense to try modifying a child's diet before treating him or her with a stimulant drug," said Dr Marvin Boris, a pediatrician in Woodbury, New York, whose 1994 study found that diet affected the behavior of two-thirds of his subjects. "Health organizations and professionals should recognize that avoiding certain foods and additives can greatly benefit some troubled children."

The difference in behaviour of school children using a dietary improvement approach can be seen from the following report by Jeffrey Smith, from the Institute for Responsible Technology, and author of "Seeds of Deception". It is taken from their newsletter on Genetically Modified foods, *Spilling the Beans*.[59]

The report overlaps into GM foods, but common sense states that ANY deviation from natural food is against the laws of our physiology, and you cannot expect to have superb health, or even normal health in many cases, if you are indulging in eating a diet that is wholly in conflict with natural living.

"Before the Appleton Wisconsin high school replaced their cafeteria's processed foods with wholesome, nutritious food, the school was described as out-of-control. There were weapons violations, student disruptions, and a cop on duty full-time. After the change in school meals, the students were calm, focused, and orderly. There were no more weapons violations, and no suicides, expulsions, dropouts, or drug violations. The new diet and improved behaviour has lasted for seven years, and now other schools are changing their meal programmes with similar results.

Years ago, a science class at Appleton found support for their new diet by conducting a cruel and unusual experiment with three mice. They fed them the junk food that kids in other high schools eat every day. The mice freaked out. Their behaviour was totally different than the three mice in the neighbouring cage. The neighbouring mice had good karma; they were fed nutritious whole foods and behaved like mice. They slept during the day inside their cardboard tube, played with each other, and acted very mouse-like.

The junk food mice, on the other hand, destroyed their cardboard tube, were no longer nocturnal, stopped playing with each other, fought often, and two mice eventually killed the third and ate it. After the three-month experiment, the students rehabilitated the two surviving junk food mice with a diet of whole foods. After about three weeks, the mice came around and acted normally.

Sister Luigi Frigo repeats this experiment every year in her second grade class in Cudahy, Wisconsin, but, mercifully, for only four days. Even on the first day of junk food, the mice's behaviour "changes drastically". They become lazy, antisocial, and nervous. And it still takes the mice about two to three weeks on unprocessed foods to return to normal. One year, the second graders tried to do the experiment again a few months later with the same mice, but this time the animals refused to eat the junk food.

Across the ocean in Holland, a student fed one group of mice genetically modified (GM) corn and soy, and another group the non-GM variety. The GM mice stopped playing with each other and withdrew into their own parts of the cage. When the student tried to pick them up, unlike their well-behaved neighbours, the GM mice scampered around in apparent fear and tried to climb the walls. One mouse in the GM group was found dead at the end of the experiment.

It's interesting to note that the junk food fed to the mice in the Wisconsin experiments also contained genetically modified ingredients. And, although the Appleton school lunch programme did not specifically attempt to remove GM foods, it happened anyway. That's because GM foods such as soy and corn and their derivatives are largely found in processed foods in America. So when the school switched to unprocessed alternatives, almost all ingredients derived from GM crops were taken out automatically.

Does this mean that GM foods negatively affect the behaviour of humans or animals? It would certainly be irresponsible to say so on the basis of a single student mice experiment and the results at Appleton. On the other hand, it is equally irresponsible to say that it doesn't."

We are just beginning to understand the influence of food on behaviour. A study in *Science* in December 2002 concluded that "food molecules act like hormones, regulating body functioning and triggering cell division.

The molecules can cause mental imbalances ranging from attention-deficit and hyperactivity disorder to serious mental illness." The problem is, we do not know which food molecules have what effect.

The bigger problem is that the composition of GM foods can change radically without our knowledge. Genetically modified foods have genes inserted into their DNA. But genes are not Legos; they don't just snap into place. Gene insertion creates unpredicted, irreversible changes. In one study, for example, a gene chip monitored the DNA before and after a single foreign gene was inserted. As much as 5 percent of the DNA's genes changed the amount of protein they were producing. Not only is that huge in itself, but these changes can multiply through complex interactions down the line.

In spite of the potential for dramatic changes in the composition of GM foods, they are typically measured for only a small number of known nutrient levels. But even if we could identify all the changed compounds, at this point we wouldn't know which might be responsible for the anti-social nature of mice or humans. Likewise, we are only beginning to identify the medicinal compounds in food. We now know, for example, that the pigment in blueberries may revive the brain's neural communication system, and the antioxidant found in grape skins may fight cancer and reduce heart disease. But what about other valuable compounds we don't know about that might change or disappear in GM varieties?

Consider GM soy. In July 1999, years after it was on the market, independent researchers published a study showing that it contains 12-14 percent less cancer-fighting phytoestrogens. What else has changed that we don't know about? [Monsanto responded with its own study, which concluded that soy's phytoestrogen levels vary too much to even carry out a statistical analysis. They failed to disclose, however, that the laboratory that conducted Monsanto's experiment had been instructed to use an obsolete method to detect phytoestrogen results.]

In 1996, Monsanto published a paper in the *Journal of Nutrition* that concluded in the title, "The composition of glyphosate-tolerant soybean seeds is equivalent to that of conventional soybeans". The study compared only a small number of nutrients and a close look at their charts revealed significant differences in the fat, ash, and carbohydrate content. In addition, GM soy meal contained 27 percent more trypsin inhibitor, a well-known soy allergen. The study also used questionable methods. Nutrient comparisons are routinely conducted on plants grown in identical conditions, so that variables such as weather and soil can be ruled out. Otherwise, differences in plant composition could be easily missed. In Monsanto's study, soybeans were planted in widely varying climates and geography.

SEXUAL ABNORMALITIES

From Louis Kuhne's *New Science of Healing* (1894):[60]

"It is an old and well-known fact to farmers, that an unnaturally increased sexual impulse among cattle is a sure sign of a disease having broken out. And it is the same with man, as anyone can observe who will look about him. I need only mention here the abnormal sexual excitement on the part of consumptives."

That fact, that sexual desire itself can be linked to illness within the body, can tie in exactly with the possibility that a health disorder in the body is behind sexual desire, even sexual perversion.

The Pottenger Cats experiment gave a wonderful insight into how far cooked diet can affect the behaviour of animals. Some of the cats fed entirely on a cooked diet displayed true homosexual behaviour, observed Pottenger. He stated:

"What is natural and what is unnatural? Rats kept in crowded captivity and fed on laboratory "balanced" food display most unnatural behaviour: they are nervous and agitated, they fight, they kill and eat their own young.[61] Cats confined in pens and fed pasteurised milk lost condition and agility and their next generation was depleted by stillbirth, miscarriage, and spontaneous abortion, with the survivors displaying many physical defects: neurosis and other abnormalities such as less anatomical differences between the sexes and homosexuality."[62]

Similar defects occurred among zoo animals. Philadelphia Zoo fed leftovers from restaurants, etc, which defects cleared after the animals' diets were changed to natural raw food.

Zoologist Desmond Morris, introducing his book *The Human Zoo* (McGraw-Hill, 1969), had this to say: "Under normal conditions, in their natural habitats, wild animals do not mutilate themselves, masturbate, attack their offspring, develop stomach ulcers, become fetishists, suffer from obesity, form homosexual pair-bonds, or commit murder. ... The zoo animals in a cage exhibit all these abnormalities that we know so well from our human comparisons. Clearly, then, the city is not a concrete jungle; it is a human zoo."

Ross Horne, M.D., in his 1997 book *Health and Survival in the 21st Century* (HarperCollins Australia), observes: "Over-sexuality is a form of neurosis, not a sign of vigour and health, and like homosexuality it is an abnormal condition which does not occur among any species of animals on Earth, including humans, when a natural environment prevails."

36.

Could You Be "Food Allergic"?

There is a strong possibility that, whatever chronic illness you may suffer from, there could be an unsuspected dietary trigger that can influence your symptoms.

It is a fact that someone could live with a chronic condition for decades and never suspect for a single moment that there could be something on the plate in front of him that will make his depression, or other condition, worse, in the next hour or so. As it is often the case that symptoms can fluctuate during the day anyway, that meal connection is extremely difficult to make, until it is pointed out.

Despite the phenomenon being known for over 50 years, it is still dismissed by mainstream medicine. This further serves to make this a poor relation in terms of public prominence.

If you experience fluctuating symptoms – they might come and go during the day – then that suggests a very high probability that there will be a food connection.

Keep a food diary for each day. Enter everything you eat or drink, with the time you start your meal and the time you finally lay down the fork, and also enter any times during the day that you observe the symptoms becoming worse. This way, a pattern can emerge. But be aware that if you smoke, your diary would need that entered as well, as cigarette smoking can be a very potent allergen.

Watch for the times your symptoms are less severe and witness if there is any worsening of your condition within half an hour to an hour after eating or drinking. Then, again, take note of the time any "reaction" wears off.

In the 1960s, there was a recognition that people with "ordinary" symptoms such as depression, or arthritis, or anxiety, or any number of others, could be "food allergic", in that many people found that their symptoms were directly linked to the meals they were eating. For example, someone who might have arthritis may find that it gets worse after eating and the symptoms abate after about one or two hours.

This recognition spawned hundreds of books on the subject of the "food allergy" condition – as it became known. Many self-help groups were set up, in the U.K. and America, despite family doctors dismissing patients' findings as "not scientific" or not proven.

Whilst medical research would not recognise the condition, it was all too real for those who found that, by manipulation of their diet, improvement could be achieved over their hated symptoms.

There are over a hundred symptoms linked to diet, but virtually any symptom of ill health, mental or physical, can be triggered by foods or substances that you can inhale or drink.

Any aspect of what you eat, drink, or inhale can be responsible for the symptoms that have perhaps plagued you for years. It is an eye-opener, and somewhat of a relief, to just make that connection, because it gives you a degree of control you might not have had prior to the discovery.

There can be confusion when setting about tracking down the culprit foods or substances. For example, some sensitive people could have an onset of their symptoms whilst walking through a department store. It would have taken a detective to work out that it was when they were passing the perfume counter, and it was the perfumes themselves that were causing the problem, and not just some random onset of their symptoms! Simply inhaling a chemical could, in some cases, trigger an attack. And only if you are constantly alert to this fact can you detect the problem substances.

Food, or chemical, allergy or sensitivity, or intolerance (all these terms are used) is almost certainly wider spread in 2012 than it was in the 1960s, by virtue of our even poorer eating habits. However, it appears the condition seems to get less exposure today than it did forty or so years ago. People seem to be even less knowledgeable of its existence today as they were then. But the syndrome is still as valid today as it ever was.

The reason why it would be problematic is easy to understand. From cigarette smoke, to eggs, to bread, to butter, to soft drinks, to alcohol, to chemicals in the kitchen – absolutely anything can trigger the symptoms. Smoking first thing in the morning, followed by a coffee, then a breakfast, then more cigarettes, then tea or coffee at work, followed by lunch and more cigarettes, means that all these things you are taking into your body are overlapping. There is no clear space, no clear dividing line, for you to assess what is happening. If everything runs into everything else, it might be difficult to make the connection.

Ideally, you would not smoke at all during a testing session. Then you would have your breakfast. You would then watch out over the next couple of hours for your symptoms to exacerbate. If they do, suspect something in your meal, or your coffee or your tea, or even your sugar. Detective work thereafter, by elimination, should find the culprit.

There are many books on detecting food/chemical allergies, but I give you my research hereunder, extracted from my book *Curing Food Allergies and Common Illnesses*, which ties in completely with the subject of this book – how your health can be improved by consuming raw foods.[63]

CHRONIC ILLNESS, FOOD "ALLERGIES" AND BODY TEMPERATURE

An intriguing observation led me on a search for the solution to my chronic illness, which started in the late 1960s. Initially considered simple fatigue, it took me several years to make a dietary link.

Thereafter, I relabelled my condition "food allergy".

I observed that, whenever I had a fever, my symptoms entirely vanished. I still had the malaise that accompanies fever, but my "food allergy" symptoms – my long-standing complaint – entirely disappeared, only to return when the fever left.

Over the next 20 years, I had three more fevers. On each occasion, without exception, my symptoms completely disappeared, but only for the duration of the fever. Surely, I thought, in fever lay the clue to the "food allergy" phenomenon.

I have also heard of other people mentioning the fever link to their illness and how they experienced relief during the period of the higher temperature. The difficulty in making the connection with your symptoms coming and going is that many people who have symptoms see them fluctuate daily, or even hourly, anyway, so if they had a fever and that coincided with relief from their symptoms, they would just see it as yet another "break" in their condition – which they experience regularly anyway.

But, as my symptoms were with me constantly, the relief I did get during fever was absolutely profound and well defined.

Visits to the library to read up on pyrexia produced no real answer. It was also clear that even the highly qualified authors did not know the true mechanism behind fever.

My own search for a solution involved over 50 fasts (water only, no food) – including two lasting a month each; four weeks on grapes only, and seven months on the Gerson therapy, as well as many other Nature Cure diets. I would abandon them all, however, because everything I ate made me ill.

I also considered that simply identifying and avoiding the problem foods was not enough. Why do some people react to ordinary foods in the first place, and not everyone? After all, if someone is "allergic" to, say, a tomato, it is not the tomato that is at fault, it is the person. Otherwise everybody would react to tomato.

FAULT "AT SITE OF SYMPTOM"

The fault surely has to lie within the person, and specifically at the site of the symptom. After all, if you have two patients with "food allergy", one might present with migraine, another with arthritis. The person with migraine will not get the arthritis and the person with arthritis will not suffer migraine. Each will have his own specific, repeating symptom in a particular part of the body. Therefore, the problem has to be at the site of the symptom.

A BLOOD FLOW PROBLEM?

Space does not permit the full explanation, but I had suspected for some years that there might be an interference in blood flow at the site of the symptom in the food allergic.

With some difficulty, I arranged to have my theory tested at the Edinburgh Royal Infirmary. I planned to get two blood flow tests, one before and one after consuming a food allergen.

Both the vascular surgeon whom I initially approached and the experienced radiologist that he recommended thought it highly unlikely that there would be a blood flow connection to my symptoms. However, they kindly allowed the testing to go ahead.

Much to the radiologist's chagrin, there was a considerable change in blood flow on the second reading, a mere half an hour after the first. His flustered response was, "But it's not scientific!" I agreed. But as it occurred after my predicting it in advance, surely the "scientific" step would have been to carry out further investigation and not just simply ignore it because it was predicted by someone not in his "field".

If, as now seemed likely, there was a hypoperfusion at the site of the symptom in the food allergic, that would give an explanation for the vast number of disorders linked to food allergy. As blood reaches every part of the body, then a reduced flow anywhere would produce symptoms anywhere in the body.

THE POSSIBILITIES

What could be causing this hypoperfusion? There could only be, I reasoned, three possibilities. Either there was something there that shouldn't be there ("something added"), or there was something not there that should be there ("something missing"), or there was damage ("something damaged"), and I included inflammation in the damaged scenario.

"Something damaged" seemed likely. But when I recalled my own dietary experiments, I had to dismiss it. My month-long fasts, which are noted for their acceleration of healing, would surely have repaired any such damage.

Besides, many food allergics can experience a severe reaction for an hour or so, then feel well after that. If there truly was damage, it wouldn't last simply an hour. Also, my seven months on a natural food diet, such diets having a long history of successful health restorations, would surely have achieved repair. But none of them did. No, I had to dismiss "something damaged" for the moment.

Then I considered "something missing". But, as I had persevered with the fruit and vegetable diet for seven months, any nutrient deficiencies would surely have been satisfied in that time. Besides, why should someone be "missing" something during the allergic reaction, yet not be an hour or so later? So "something missing" was shelved for the moment.

"Something added" looked the likeliest culprit. Space does not allow me a full explanation, but I initially favoured old drug or chemical residues in the system. However, my fasting and natural food attempts, both famous for the elimination of toxins, had failed to remove them.

And, if an old drug residue was responsible, why should the problem only occur for an hour or so, then vanish? How could it change shape or form to create a blood flow blockage in that hour and then settle down?

214

Also, as old drugs and chemicals become adipose-bound, how could they create an interference with the blood flow?

And why should my symptoms disappear only when I had a fever, if old drugs or chemicals were the reason? But the best reason for dismissing old drugs and chemicals was when I recalled that arthritis, a classic food allergy disorder, has been around for centuries. Modern drugs have not.

So, "something added" it must be. But what? After dispelling drugs and other toxins, I arrived at the astonishing conclusion that perhaps the "something added" might be LIVING! In other words, a parasite.

Parasites tend to settle in the lumen of blood vessels. That would explain how they could interfere with blood flow. Perhaps simple obstruction in the micro-circulation by hordes of these creatures is all it takes to produce symptoms.

PARASITE SYMPTOMS

I wanted to know how many symptoms attributable to "food allergy" could be caused by parasites. Trawling through the parasitology literature, I uncovered the following catalogue of symptoms regularly found listed in food allergy books:

Symptoms Potentially Associated with Food Allergies

Asthma	Mouth ulcers	Skin infections
Rheumatic fever	Depression	Warts
Arthritis	Personality changes	Abdominal pain
Hyperactivity/ADD	Chronic fatigue	Burning pain in penis on
Alzheimer's	Bloating	urination
Epilepsy	Conjunctivitis	Jaundice
Headaches	Oedema	Hepatitis
Mental confusion	Eczema	Anaemia
Urticaria	Osteomyelitis	High blood pressure
Nervousness	Cystitis	Heartbeat, irregular
Migraine	Irritable bowel syndrome (IBS)	(arrhythmia)
Weight loss	Sore throats	Myalgia
Weight gain	Impetigo	Dermatitis
Vascular disorders	Acne	Urinary tract infections
Thrush		Anorexia

In case you may think that "simple blockage" by parasites may be too lowly an explanation for a chronic illness capable of baffling science for years, let me quote from the 1999 edition of *Modern Parasitology*:

"Both lymphatic and ocular filariasis are accompanied by gross pathological changes, elephantiasis and blindness, but it is not clear if these have any immunological basis and current opinion favours simple obstruction."

So, despite all their investigations into the subject, these parasitologists only as recently as 1999 are recognising that simple blockage by parasites may hold the key to an illness that had long baffled them.

I FLY TO CALIFORNIA

I found someone else homing in on the parasite connection to ill health. Dr Hulda Clark, of California, a former government-funded scientist, claims that parasites are implicated in a huge number of chronic disorders, including cancers. I flew out to her clinic and was taught the rudiments of her electronic method of testing for parasites. I took the opportunity to have my sputum tested for their presence. It was positive for several parasite species! Since that time I have learned how to examine microscopically my own blood, sputum, urine and faeces for parasites.

Being told you have parasites is one thing, actually seeing them for yourself coming out of your body is quite another! I took photographs using a photomicrographic camera, at 100x magnification, Lugol stained, showing parasite eggs to which I had unwittingly been host.

ELIMINATION OF PARASITES

Parasites are all around us. A newspaper of 29th November 1998 stated that one baby cereal tested contained over 20,000 mites per kilo!

In separate research, a sample of six types of vegetable in an American study, carried out between 1979 and 1981, showed that parasite eggs are virtually everywhere. It showed that over 50% of all vegetables tested had some parasites.

Nematodes are human parasites that are extremely abundant in nature. A single spadeful of garden soil may contain a million or more!

Dr Clark was attempting to eliminate parasites by using herbs and instructing her patients to avoid parasite eggs by scrupulously removing all dirt from fruits and vegetables. She also recommends boiling milk and washing vegetables in an iodine solution to kill Ascaris eggs; sterilising your toothbrush with grain alcohol each time you use it; and not licking your fingers turning over pages in a book. Despite these and more measures, many patients would still harbour parasites.

But surely this approach was missing something? Watch any nature programme and you will see tigers tearing open their prey and inevitably consuming dirt. It seems to be perfectly natural. Yet wild tigers are strong and healthy beasts that do not get food allergies or cancers.

And what about those people who do not wash their fruits and vegetables or boil their milk? What about those people who do not sterilise their toothbrush? What about those people who do lick their fingers turning over pages? Not all become ill. It is clear that many people must be taking in these parasites, yet remain well.

No, simply trying to avoid every single parasite and every single egg for the rest of your life cannot be the entire answer; they are so prevalent, it would be impossible to do so. There had to be another way.

YOUR "INTERNAL ENVIRONMENT"

It seemed logical to consider that the person's health, his/her "internal environment" if you will, had to play a part in the equation. After all, it is well known in gardening that plant parasites do not attack healthy plants.

If that is the case, the only way to improve the health of a patient is to improve his/her diet dramatically.

THE DISCOVERY

I obtained 50 million insect parasitic nematodes, *Steinernema feltiae*, in an attempt to study their behaviour.

I noted that they would respond whenever the microscope's sub-stage illuminator was switched on. But, other than that, I was floundering to capture any other significant aspect of their functioning.

One day, I read that, when amoebas are studied on a slide, if one end is cooled and the other end of the slide is warmed, these parasites will migrate to the warm end.

Amoebas are parasites capable of producing much illness in man. Amoebic dysentery is an illness caused by the organism *Entamoeba histolytica* and is spread by contaminated food, water, or flies. If the organism enters the portal circulation, amoebic abscess can result. These abscesses can also invade the lung, brain, or spleen.

I read on for a while, then stopped. I had just read something that appeared insignificant at first, but suddenly hit me like a sledgehammer. If the parasitic amoebas on the microscope slide responded to temperature change, here, therefore, was an absolutely vital clue to their behaviour:

Parasites are *TEMPERATURE-SENSITIVE*!

Therefore, if my personal food allergy condition was linked to parasites, and if parasites are influenced by temperature, then that explains why my food allergy symptoms disappeared when I had a fever. The low body temperature that I knew I had, but paid little attention to, must have been ideal for the parasites and they were only overcome when my body temperature increased.

LOW BODY TEMPERATURE

It was also only a relatively recent discovery that I had a chronic low body temperature, generally in the low 97s (degrees Fahrenheit).

Perhaps if we could raise our core body temperature, that would keep us parasite-free? Indeed, food allergy free? But how?

I then recalled that, in *Cures that Work*, a founder member of Tyringham Health Clinic had recovered from hypothyroidism, which would have involved subnormal body temperature, by sustaining a natural food diet for over a year. By dietary means, she must surely have managed to raise her body temperature.

I also recalled my seven-month diet on fruits and vegetables. My body temperature, which I recorded each morning, was erratically, but inexorably, climbing. However, I had never charted it.

I decided to check back on my diary and do just that. The overall climb in temperature was undeniable. However, I had not sustained it for the full 18 months to 2/3 years. The number of days of 97.8°F or above was increasing as the diet progressed, and the number of days on the lower level of 97.5°F and below had all but disappeared.

Researchers Emanuel Donchin and Noel Marshall, from the University of Chicago, found that slight low body temperature, just one or two degrees below normal, was enough to reduce certain brain responses in test subjects.

Dr Stephen Langer estimates that 40% of Americans have subnormal temperatures. He found that a mere one degree below the desired 98.6°F is sufficient to produce a host of mental and physical symptoms such as headaches, depression, nervousness, etc.

Hospital blood tests for thyroid function are unreliable. Extreme cases might be picked up, but many people will have a sub-clinical thyroid system malfunction, which will be missed by these tests, as they gauge glandular function by measuring levels of thyroid hormones in the bloodstream. But the thyroid hormones have their action in the cells of the body at the nuclear membrane receptors, and there is no method of accurately measuring such intracellular activity.

CANCER

The parasite link to body temperature would explain why so many recoveries from cancer and other chronic diseases occur on natural food diets like the Gerson therapy.

It is not only Dr Clark who has implicated parasites in cancer. Only as recently as 1999, Professor Jan Walbloomers, of the Free University in Amsterdam, found that the HPV, or human papilloma virus, exists in over 99.7% of cases of cervical cancer. This is the first real evidence that parasites do exist in cancer. That would now give a better explanation for the success of the Gerson therapy, as the diet would surely raise the body temperature of such patients, overwhelming the micro-organisms.

ONE DEGREE ENOUGH?

The question is often asked, "How can a mere one degree affect parasites to the extent that it can incapacitate them?"

Nature already employs heat as a means of defending our bodies against micro-organisms. At such times of infection, she produces fever in the body to overcome them. And when you consider that fever is 100°F, just over one degree above 98.6°F, then clearly Nature herself considers one degree sufficient to defeat them.

Besides, it is our human measuring that dictates that one degree is one degree. If microscopic organisms were to use their own measuring standards, I am sure our "mere" one degree would translate into a thousand of their degrees!

SCIENTIFIC CONFIRMATION

I then found medical confirmation that micro-organisms can be directly killed by fever in the host animal. From *Pyretics and Antipyretics*:

"It has been recognised that syphilis (caused by the parasite Treponema pallidum) and gonorrhoea (caused by the parasite Neisseria gonorrhoea) are heat sensitive and are killed directly by increasing the temperature of the victim. Indeed, before the advent of antibiotics, treatment used to consist of using injections in order to bring about artificial fevers."

And, recognising the existing lack of precise knowledge on parasites, *Microbial and Parasitic Infection* quotes:

"A pathogen must be able to multiply in or on the host's tissues. This means that the host's tissues must supply appropriate nutrients, atmospheric conditions and temperature for the pathogen's growth ..."

Pyretics and Antipyretics states:

"The question of the beneficial value of fever has been the subject of speculation for many years. Fevers could be beneficial to an animal in two ways:

The high body temperatures of fever could exceed the temperature beyond which the infectious micro-organism could live and thereby directly kill it.

Indirectly by affecting one or several biochemical, cellular or humoral components of the body which in turn destroy the micro-organism."

LONG-LIVED ORGANISMS

Human parasites are extremely long-lived. Strongyloides can remain in the system for up to 30 years and *Taenia saginata* – beef tapeworms – can live in humans for up to 25 years.

Ascaris lumbricoides is the commonest parasite on the planet and it is estimated that approximately one billion people have the worm.

Asthma has been linked to *Ascaris* after laboratory workers studying them developed the condition – yet further evidence of the allergy link to micro-organisms.

Parasites vary in size, from worms several feet long down to the smallest of all, viruses.

WHY PARASITES HAVE BEEN OVERLOOKED

Could micro-organisms be responsible for a host of common health disorders, yet simply be overlooked? Almost certainly.

If medical science can miss something as highly visible and obvious as a chunk of bread and cheese as being responsible for someone's symptoms – and it has – is it not reasonable that they could similarly miss something that is invisible to the naked eye, hidden inside the body, and undetectable by X-ray or MRI equipment?

But the main reason could be the confusion over what are harmless (commensal) and harmful (pathogenic) parasites.

The *Color Atlas and Textbook of Diagnostic Parasitology* states: "Few people realize that only a few decades ago *Giardia lamblia*, now recognized as the leading cause of intestinal parasitic infections in the United States, was not considered a pathogen."

Now, there is confusion over the status of *Blastocystis hominis*. Next to yeast, *Blastocystis hominis* is the most frequently observed organism in faecal samples.

Also, many people can harbour *Giardia lamblia* or *Entamoeba histolytica* and not display symptoms; whilst symptoms from what were considered harmless commensal parasites, *Entamoeba coli* or *Endolimax nana*, have been reported.

I suggest that "commensal" parasites are misclassified, because of the complication that is inherent in food allergy.

With food allergics, if parasites truly are implicated, their activity would occur only for the duration of the reaction. At such time they could be declared pathogenic. But the same parasite, once the reaction wore off and was no longer causing symptoms, could be declared a harmless commensal: that cause for misclassification would occur if the test subjects had masked (hidden) food allergies.

And what if the subjects were not food allergics? The parasite this time would appear a harmless commensal. But it would only be harmless to that non-food-allergic person. To the food-allergic patient, that harmless parasite could well be a pathogen. Just as a slice of bread may be harmless to a non-food-allergic, to a food allergic, that same bread may be harmful.

It is clear that we should not be trying to establish the "pathogenicity" of any particular organism, but rather assess the health of the patient. After all, people can "carry" a parasite, yet be entirely asymptomatic; whilst others can be at death's door with the same organism. HIV and meningitis organisms are such examples.

Classifying micro-organisms into their pathogenicity or non-pathogenicity is a misleading exercise. The missing factor that separates the ill from the well might well be simple body temperature, now that we see its importance in the life of the human parasite.

From *Microbial and Parasitic Infection*:

"Failure of the host's defences to eliminate a pathogen soon after its arrival may result in persistent active disease. Often, however, there is a balance between the pathogen and the defences, and the infection may remain asymptomatic for many years, but turn into active disease again when the balance is shifted in favour of the pathogen."

The same book later states: "An increase in body temperature is a very common host response to infection. It may well be protective in some circumstances, e.g. by providing an environment too warm for optimal growth of the pathogen [micro-organism]."

HEREDITARY ILLNESS: THE ANSWER?

The well-known tendency for allergies to "run in the family" might now be explained.

We know that "allergic" conditions can be inherited. But the real truth could well be that, as parasites are involved in allergic activity, it is the parasitic organisms themselves that may be passed to the offspring from the parents.

37.

Do We Need Chemicals On Our Food?

Our farmers have somehow been convinced that it is essential that we have all our crops and fields sprayed with toxic chemicals. Such is the skill of the chemical industry in selling its wares.

It has somehow been forgotten that fruits and vegetables have survived and thrived for millions of years without the need for that industry or its products.

Organic foods, given no spraying whatsoever, are not only healthier plants, but are free from toxic chemicals that would otherwise be consumed with the fruit or vegetables.

Farmers have been won over by all the impressive "spin" given to them in sales pitches – that the crops could fail unless they are sprayed with that industry's poisons.

I am no farmer, but I reiterate: fruits and vegetables have survived and thrived for millions of years without the need for this comparatively new industry's toxic products sprayed over our children's food.

If these plants hadn't survived and thrived, they would simply not be in existence today. But they *are* in existence today, which *proves* Nature is more than capable of looking after her own, without any need from global chemical giants' products.

The growing success of organic foods is evidence itself that chemicals are not needed.

The intelligent reader who has come thus far will realise that the natural and bountiful soil on the likes of the Marquesa Islands, and other areas where healthy societies lived, was completely natural and free from chemical interference. To compare such beautiful soils to our intensively-farmed lands of today should provide evidence in itself as to the reason for man's increasing poor state of health.

Would the Marquesa or other islanders' health be the same if they were fed food grown on soil heavily sprayed with chemicals? Clearly not, as the world-famous Rodale Institute's 30-year study on the comparison between natural (organic) farming and intensive chemical farming shows.

The Rodale Institute recently – in September 2011 – announced the results of the Farming Systems Trial, America's longest-running side-by-side comparison of organic and conventional farming practices.[64] Originally created to study the transition from conventional to organic production, this 30-year study also examined productivity, soil quality, energy, and economics.

Key findings show:

- Organic yields match or surpass conventional yields.
- Organic yields outperform conventional yields in years of drought.
- Organic farming systems build rather than deplete soil organic matter, making it a more sustainable system.
- Organic farming uses 45 percent less energy and is more efficient.
- Conventional agricultural systems produce 40 percent more greenhouse gases.
- Organic farming systems are more profitable than conventional farming systems.

After 30 years of a rigorous side-by-side comparison, the Institute confidently concludes that organic methods are improving the quality of our food, the health of our soils and water, and the conditions of our nation's rural areas. Organic agriculture creates more jobs, provides a liveable income for farmers, and can restore America's confidence in our farming community and food system.

"America's farming techniques affect the health of our families, our communities, and our planet. The Farming Systems Trial shows that organic farming is the healthiest and safest way to feed the world, provide much-needed jobs, reduce our greenhouse gas emissions, and protect precious natural resources," says Mark Smallwood, Executive Director of the Rodale Institute.

Dr Elaine Ingham, Chief Scientist at Rodale Institute, states:

"The Farming Systems Trial clearly documents in a replicated, scientific fashion, that many of the current myths are not true. Organic agriculture does not result in the grower losing money, does not result in lower yields, or more expensive management practices. The next step forward is to educate growers, whether they are conventional or organic, in the methods used in the Farming Systems Trial, to assure equal or better yields through farming practices that do not harm the environment."

The trial is slanted to continue with a new focus on nutrition and human health. "We have shown that organic can feed the world. Now it is time to take on the matter of feeding the world well," said Smallwood.

REFERENCES

1   NewsWithViews.com, 20th February, 2005.

2   Johns Hopkins University, School of Public Health: *Chronic Conditions: Making the Case for Ongoing Care.* September, 2004.

3   Horne, Ross, *Health and Survival in the 21st Century.* Australia. 1997.

4   Wulzen and Wagtendonk, Oregon State University: *Ann. Rheum. Dis.*, 9(2): 97-108, June 1950.

5   Kouchakoff, Dr Paul, Institute of Clinical Chemistry, Lausanne, Switzerland: *The Influence of Food Cooking on the Blood Formula of Man.* Proceedings: First International Congress of Microbiology, Paris, 1930.

6   Olsen, Gwen: *Confessions of an Rx Drug Pusher.* iUniverse Star, New York, 2009.

7   Bircher-Benner, R.: *Raw Food in Health and Disease.* The Vegetarian Society, 1947.

8   Friedrich and Peters: "Treatment of Cirrhosis of the Liver with Raw Food". *Med. Wochenschr.*, 86, 453-455, 1939.

9   Kanai, I.: "Effect of Vegetarian Diet, Raw or Cooked, on Oxidation in the Body". *Stchr. E.D. Ges. Exp. Med.*, 89, 131-140, 1933.

10 Hawkins, H. F.: "Raw Foods Help Prevent Pyorrhea". *Let's Live*, 3rd April, 1955.

11 Hanke, M. T.: *Diet and Dental Health.* Chicago, University of Chicago Press, 1933.

12 Chaney, G.: "Rapid Healing of Peptic Ulcers in Patients Receiving Fresh Cabbage Juice". *California Medicine*, 70: 10-14, 1949.

13 Birnberg, T. L.: "Raw Apple Diet in the Treatment of Diarrheal Conditions in Children". *Amer. J. Dis. Child*, 45, 18-24, 1933.

14 Gaisbauer, M. and Langosch, A.: "Raw Food and Immunity". *Fortschr Med.*, 10: 108(17): 338-40, June, 1990.

15 Nenonen, M. T., Helve, T. A., Rauma, A. L., and Hanninen, O. O.:

"Uncooked, lactobacilli-rich, vegan food and rheumatoid arthritis". *British Journal of Rheumatology*, 37(3): 274-281, March 1998.

16 Johns Hopkins University, School of Public Health: *Chronic Conditions: Making the Case for Ongoing Care.* September, 2004.

17 Pottenger, Dr Francis, Jr: *Pottenger's Cats: A Study in Nutrition.* Price-Pottenger Nutrition Foundation, 2009.

18 McCann, Alfred W.: *Science of Eating: How to Insure Stamina, Endurance, Vigor, Strength and Health in Infancy, Youth and Age.* George H. Doran Company, New York, 1919.

19 Taylor, John: Pamphlet: *The Old, Old, Very Old Man or the Age and Long Life of Thomas Parr.* 1635.

20 McCarrison, R.: *Studies in Deficiency Diseases.* London, Oxford University Press, 1921.

21 Fink, H. and Schlie, I.: "Skimmed Milk Acquires the Property of Producing Liver Necrosis During the Drying Process". *Inst. Garungswiss. Phil.*, 45, 21-22, 1955.

22 Hess, A. E.: "Infantile Scurvy, V.A. Study of Its Pathogenesis." *Am. J. Dis. Child*, November, 1917.

23 Sprawson, E.: "Raw Milk and Sound Teeth". *Pub. Health*, 47, 388-395, 1934.

24 Steiner, O.: "Treatment of Milk". *Levensmitteluntersuch u. Hyg.,* 94-103, 1933.

25 Cohen, C. H. and Ruelle, G.: "Plea in Favor of Raw Milk". *Rev. Franc, de Pediat.*, 8: 312-323, 1932.

26 Fisher, R. A. and Bartlett, S.: "Pasteurised and Raw Milk". *Nature,* 127: 591-592, 1931.

27 Perkin, M. R. and Strachan, D. P.: *The Journal of Allergy and Clinical Immunology*, 117 (6): 1374-81, 2006.

28 Pottenger, F. M. and Simonsen, D. G.: "Deficient Calcification Produced by Diet: Experimental and Clinical Considerations". *Transactions Am. Ther. Soc.*, 39, 1939.

29 Kirkpatrick, G.: "Raw Milk Versus Pasteurised Milk". Seattle. *Nat. Nutrition League*, 1950.

30 Scott, Dr Ernest and Erf, Prof Lowell: "Rat Studies with Raw and Pasteurised Milk". *Jersey Bulletin,* 50: 210-211; 224-226, 237, 1950.

31 International School of Orthopathy. Dr Herbert Shelton and Dr George Clements, 1963.

32 Densmore, Emmet, M.D.: *How Nature Heals.* Swan Sonnenschein

& Co., London, 1892.

33 Source: *Gastroenterology*, 2011; DOI; 10.153.

34 Bishop, Beata: *A Time to Heal – Triumph Over Cancer.* Penguin Books.

35 Gerson, Max, M.D.: *A Cancer Therapy: Results of Fifty Cases.* Gerson Institute, 1958.

36 Gerson, Charlotte and Walker, Morton: *The Gerson Therapy: The Proven Nutritional Program for Cancer and Other Illnesses.* New York, Kensington Publishing Corporation.

37 Lechner, P. and Kronberger, L.: "Experience with the use of dietary therapy in surgical oncology". *Atkuelle Ernaehrungsmedin*, 2: 15, 1990.

38 Wheatley, Carmen: *Living Proof: The Case of the .005% Survivor – A Medical Scrutiny*. Scribner, 2002. ISBN 0-7432-0677-0.

39 Hoshino, Y. (Title in Japanese), 1998. ISBN 4-8376-1096-X.

40 Nolfi, Dr Kristine: *My Adoption of a Raw Food Diet and My Breast Cancer.* Originally published around 1950.

41 Sun, Dr Wong Hon: *How I Overcame Inoperable Cancer.* Exposition Press, New York, 1975.

42 CureZone: *Educating Instead of Medicating*. June, 2005. Website: curezone.com.

43 Ferrante, Frank and Cafe Gratitude, Los Angeles. Calif. Film: *May I be Frank?* Website: mayibefrankmovie.com.

44 Clements, Dr George and Shelton, Dr Herbert: International School of Orthopathy.

45 Holmes, Dr Oliver Wendell: *Medical Essays*, p.260.

46 Howenstine, Dr James. Website: NewsWithViews.com, February, 2005.

47 BBC News, 7th January, 2005.

48 WDDTY (What Doctors Don't Tell You): Vol. 21, Issue 8, 2011.

49 WDDTY (What Doctors Don't Tell You): Newsletter, 11th August, 2011.

50 NaturalBias.com. Vin Miller: "Biased and Deceitful Research", 12th October, 2009.

51 Citizens Commission on Human Rights International, December, 2011.

52 Wikipedia: List of Withdrawn Drugs. Website: wikipedia.org.

53 Gislason, Dr Gunnar: *Non-steroidal Anti-inflammatory Drugs*. Results of 8-year study. Gentofte University Hospital, 2010.

54   Source: *Gastroenterology*, 2011; DOI; 10.153.

55   *Natural Life Magazine*: May/June, 1996.

56   *The Sunday Times*, 29th August, 2010.

57   World Health Organisation stats. Source: wikipedia.org.

58   Price, Weston: *Nutrition and Physical Degeneration*. Keats Publishing, 2003.

59   Smith, Jeffrey: "Seeds of Deception". Report taken from *Spilling the Beans* newsletter, from Institute of Responsible Technology,1st September, 2004.

60   Kuhne, Louis: *New Science of Healing*. 1894.

61   Fox, Dr H.: *Disease in Captive Wild Animals and Birds*. J. B. Lippincott, Philadelphia, PA, 1923.

62   Pottenger, Dr Francis: *The Effect of Heat Processed Foods and Pasteurized Vitamin D Milk on the Dentofacial Structures of Experimental Animals*. 1946.

63   Hunter, Alan: *Curing Food Allergies and Common Illnesses*. Ashgrove Press, 2000.

64   Rodale Institute: *Farming Systems Trial*. 16th September, 2011.

INDEX

chopping/ grating 94–5
Christian, F. 163
chronic fatigue, as possible food allergy symptom 212, 215
chronic illness
    defined 23
    statistics 23
    vs acute conditions 9
cigarettes/ smoking
    and food allergies/ blockages 211–12
    long-term effects of 33–4
    nicotine and heart complaints 90
    poisonousness of 90, 93
'circular reasoning' in science 142
cirrhosis 17–18
Clark, Dr H. 216
Clark, Dr J. 81
Clements, Dr G. 54, 108
clinical trials 76, 86, 124–6
cocktails of drugs, effects 61–2, 66–8
coeliac disease 16
colds 92
Coleman, Dr V. 68
colloidal minerals 6, 20
'comfort food' 107
commensal parasites 221
Confessions of an Rx Drug Pusher (Olsen, 2009) 9, 121
conjunctivitis, as possible food allergy symptom 215
constipation 20
constitutional effects of raw diet 17, 22, 90–1
consumption *see* tuberculosis (TB/ consumption)
'contagious' disease 140–4
Cook, Captain J. 152, 171, 173–4
cooking foods
    and anaemia 18
    destruction of nutrients 33–5, 190, 193–4
    for food 'safety' 1
    harmlessness of cooked food myth 34–5
    history of 33–5
    hormones destroyed by heating 7
    oxidation, impaired by cooked foods 18
    Polynesian cooking methods 194
    temperature (of cooking), importance of 52
Coppinger, R.W. 172–3
corruption in medicine 'industry' 119–20
cot death, and vaccination 134–5
cream, raw, 'anti-stiffness' chemical 7
cures, medical profession not finding 2–3, 5, 9, 62
CureZone 101–2
Cushing's Syndrome 82
cystitis, as possible food allergy symptom 215

Daniels, A.L. 52
Davidson, J. 105
Davison, J. 77
Day, Dr L. 105
de Vries, A. 31–2
dead food vs live food 89, 90
Denman, L. 54–9
Dent, M. 82
dental arch formation 25, 50, 145, 173, 175, 177, 180
dental health
    in animal studies 45
    Gerson therapy 85
    gum disease 19
    Pottenger Cats study 25
    Price, Dr Weston A. 145–6, 174, 177, 194
    in 'primitive' societies 157, 175, 177, 180
    and raw/ pasteurised milk 48
depression 197, 215
dermatitis, as possible food allergy symptom 215
diabetes 76, 82, 85
diarrhoea
    and raw/ pasteurised milk 49
    'scraped raw apple' diet 20
diclofenac 129–30
digestion
    raw food easier on 90–1
    and raw/ pasteurised milk 49
digestive leukocytosis 7–8, 144

'disease', definitions of 112–14
dogs
    fed on refined flour 31
    fresh meat vs processed food 46
Donchin, E. 218
Dose, H.F. 183, 186
dried fruit 93
drug industry
    drug testing 62–3
    and 'evidence-based' medicine 121,
    122
    immunity from prosecution 129
    influence over medical training 2,
    117
    influencing research 117–23
    profits threatened by nutritional
    approaches 8
    responsible for researching their own
    products 123
    safety of prescription drugs 124–31
drugs
    cocktails of drugs, effects 66–8,
    130–1
    damage caused by prescribed drugs
    (iatrogenesis) 68
    don't restore health or cure 68
    drug poisoning child death story
    68–9
    list of withdrawn drugs 125–6
    progression of development 116
    toxicity of 61–2, 89–90, 101

eczema 49, 215
Eddie, Dr E.S. 29–30
Effexor (venlafaxine) 124
eggs
    allergic reaction to (supposed) 202–3
    raw 97
emphysema 80
enzymes 6–7, 198
epilepsy, as possible food allergy symptom
215
Eppinger, H. 17
Erf, Prof L. 51
Evers, Dr J. 15
'evidence-based' medicine 121, 122,
124–31

Ewarts, H.W. 50
excretion 90
exercise 97–100

facial changes 16, 25, 173
Farming Systems Trial 224
Ferrante, F. 106–7
fertilisers 34, 90
fever *see also* body temperature
    benefits of 220
    link to food allergies 212–13
Fiji islanders 176
filtrate-factor, of vegetables 7
Finch, Captain 155–6
Fink, H. 46
First Medical Clinic of the University of
Vienna 17
fish
    eating eyes of 192
    fish liver 98
    raw fish 150
    seafood in 'primitive' diets 173, 176
Fisher, Dr 49
'five zones of influence' 16–17
Folk, Dr. 45
food allergies 49, 197–208, 210–22
Food and Drug Administration (FDA)
123, 124
food diaries 202, 210
Food Hospital (UK C4 TV programme) 2,
118
Foord, Dr A. 27
Forster, Dr 171
Forsythe, J. 78–9
Foust, E.C. 46
Franks, L.W. 50
Fredricks, C. 80
freshness of food 193
Friedrich, Dr 17
Frigo, Sr L. 206
fruit
    5 a day recommendation 104
    dried fruit 93
    grape cures 19
    not mixing with vegetables 94
    pineapple juice 96

Hunza people 3, 43–6, 194
hydrophilic colloids 20
hyperactivity 203, 206, 215
hyperpofusion 214

iatrogenesis 68
immunity 63, 77
impetigo, as possible food allergy
symptom 215
'infectious' diseases 140–4
Ingham, Dr E. 224
internal environment 217
irradiated milk 49
irritable bowel syndrome (IBS) 215

Jagadisan, T. 119–20
Japanese diet vs American diet 104
jaundice 44, 215
Jones, M.R. 176
juices *see also* Gerson therapy
    cabbage juice 20
    carrot juice 12
    hot juices 98
    pineapple juice 96
    for treating TB 11–12
    vegetable juices recommended by UK
    Ministry of Health 18
'Jungborn' clinic 12–13
Just, A. 13

Kanai, I. 18
Kaunitz, H. 17
Kennedy, J. 80
Kinderheilk, J.F. 18
King, Captain 175
Kirkpatrick, Dr 50
Kirschner, Dr H.E. 11
Kitchin, P.C. 52
Koehn, C.J. 46
Kouchakoff, Dr P. 8, 144
Kraft, R.A. 45
Kronprinz Willem sailors 115–16, 138,
140–1
Krusenstern, Captain 153
Kuhne, L. 208
Kuratsune, Dr M. 18

Langer, Dr S. 218
Langsdorff, G .von 153–4
Larsen, N.P. 176
Lechner, Dr P. 86
Lemly, M. 80
Lennox, A. 83
'Let Food be thy Medicine' 118
leukocytosis 7–8, 144
lifespan, extending 36–8, 108–11, 148
Lind, J. 115
live food vs dead food 89, 90
liver (raw)
    and animals 46
    as treatment for cancer 96–7
    as treatment for pernicious anaemia
    12
liver cirrhosis 17–18
Loughlin, R. 52
Ludd, M. 50

MacDonald, Dr 13–14
Madeira-Mamore railway workers 182–8
Madsen, N.P. 50–1
Magendie, F. 46
Marianas islanders 177–8
Marquesa islanders 149–60
Marshall, N. 218
Mattick, E. 52
May I be Frank (film) 107
McCandlish, A. 52–3
McCann, A. 29, 141, 182
McCarrison, Sir R. 3, 42, 43–6
McCay, Dr C. 46
McClure, Dr F.J. 45
McFarland, R.D. 52
meat, raw 12 *see also* liver (raw); pork;
beef
media blackouts on natural health stories
122–3
medical science, progress of 115–16
medical training
    doesn't cover nutrition 2
    influence of pharma industry 2, 117
medication, stopping 10
Melanesian people 176–7
melanoma 81, 85
Melville, H. 156–7

Reynolds, Dr W.E. 112
rheumatic fever 50, 215
Richet, Prof C. 12
rickets 48–9
Rodale Institute 224
rofecoxib (Vioxx) 123, 127
root vegetables 56, 89
rosiglitazone (Avandia) 121
Russell, Dr J.F. 1

Sabatino, Dr F. 5
Sabin, Dr 137–8
salt 17, 193
Samoan society 176
Sampson, Dr. 180
Sandler, Dr B.P. 137
Sanford, Dr C. 46
Sauerbruch, Dr F. 76
Scheibner, Dr V. 136
Schlie, I. 46
Schmidt-Nielson, S. S. 52
school meals 205
Schreiber, Dr V. 134
Schweitzer, A. 76, 77
Science of Eating, The (McCann, 1918)
29, 31–2, 182
Scott, Dr E. 51
'scraped raw apple' diet 20
scurvy
    and animal/ fish flesh 192
    discovery of 115
    and milk 47–8
selective capacity, of cells 17
self-healing 60–70, 99, 112, 113
senility, absent in animals 39
Sex Life of Wild Animals, The (Burns,
1953) 65
sexual abnormalities 208–9
Shackleton, B. 20, 200
Shelton, Dr H. 2–3, 9, 54, 62, 69, 74, 116
Shive, Dr W. 20
SIDS, and vaccination 134–5
Simms, H.D. 7
Simpson, Dr G.C. 29–30
single meal a day diet 96–100
skin infections, as possible food allergy
symptom 215

Smallwood, M. 224
Smith, Dr L. 183
Smith, J. 205
smoking *see* cigarettes
soil deficiencies 34, 90, 190
sore throats, as possible food allergy
symptom 215
South Sea Islanders 29
soy, GM 207
spices 193
splenic leukaemia, carrot juice treatment
of 12
Sprawson, Dr E. 48
statistics, relative vs absolute 101
Steiner, Dr O. 45, 49
Stevenson, R.L. 159
Strachan, D.P. 49
sugar 193
sugar cane 150
swine flu vaccine 133

Tahitian islanders 170–3
Takayasu's Arteritis (pulseless disease)
81–2
tamoxifen 101–2
Taylor, Liz 68
temperature (of body) *see* body
temperature
temperature (of cooking), importance of
52
'terminator genes' 120
Thalidomide 122, 124–5, 128
Thompson, Sir A.J. 39
thrush, as possible food allergy symptom
215
thyroid functioning tests 219
Time to Heal, A (Bishop, 2005) 75, 105
Tongan society 173–4
Torres Strait islanders 177
Tristan da Cunha islanders 179–80
tuberculosis (TB/ consumption)
    beef juice treatment 12
    and beri-beri 186
    bovine TB 139–40, 142–4
    and Dr Max Gerson 58–9, 76
    no pharmaceutical cure yet for 1, 7
    on Polynesian islands 159

238

Lightning Source UK Ltd.
Milton Keynes UK
UKHW020731070622
404062UK00006B/342

9 780755 207404